Adolescent Sexual Behavior and Childbearing

T0234271

Developmental Clinical Psychology and Psychiatry Series

Series Editor: Alan E. Kazdin, Yale University

Recent volumes in this series . . .

Adolescent Sexual Behavior and Childbearing

Laurie Schwab Zabin
Sarah C. Hayward

Volume 26.
Developmental Clinical Psychology and Psychiatry

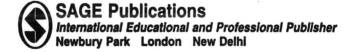
SAGE Publications
International Educational and Professional Publisher
Newbury Park London New Delhi

For information address:

SAGE Publications, Inc.
2455 Teller Road
Newbury Park, California 91320

SAGE Publications Ltd.
6 Bonhill Street
London EC2A 4PU
United Kingdom

SAGE Publications India Pvt. Ltd.
M-32 Market
Greater Kailash I
New Delhi 110 048 India

Printed in the United States of America

Library of Congress Cataloging-in-Publication Data

Zabin, Laurie Schwab.
    Adolescent sexual behavior and childbearing / Laurie Schwab Zabin.
Sarah C. Hayward.
        p. cm. —(Developmental clinical psychology and psychiatry:
    v. 26)
    Includes bibliographical references and index.
    ISBN 0-8039-4258-3 (cl).—ISBN 0-8039-4259-1 (pb)
        1. Teenage pregnancy—United States. 2. Teenagers—United States—
    Sexual behavior. 3. Birth control—United States. I. Hayward,
    Sarah C. II. Title. III. Series.
    HQ759.4.Z34   1993
    306,7'0835—dc20   92-35508

94 95 96 10 9 8 7 6 5 4 3 2

Sage Production Editor: Diane S. Foster

CONTENTS

SERIES EDITOR'S INTRODUCTION

Interest in child development and adjustment is by no means new. Yet only recently has the study of children benefitted from advances in both clinical and scientific research. Advances in the social and biological sciences, the emergence of disciplines and subdisciplines that focus exclusively on childhood and adolescence, and greater appreciation of the impact of such influences as the family, peers, and school have helped accelerate research on developmental psychopathology. Apart from interest in the study of child development and adjustment for its own sake, the need to address clinical problems of adulthood naturally draws one to investigate precursors in childhood and adolescence.

Within a relatively brief period, the study of psychopathology among children and adolescents has proliferated considerably. Several different professional journals, annual book series, and handbooks devoted entirely to the study of children and adolescents and their adjustment document the proliferation of work in the field. Nevertheless there is a paucity of resource material that presents information in an authoritative, systematic, and disseminable fashion. The field needs to convey the latest developments and to represent different disciplines, approaches, and conceptual views to the topics of childhood and adolescent adjustment and maladjustment.

The Sage Series on **Developmental Clinical Psychology and Psychiatry** is designed to serve uniquely several needs of the field. The series encompasses individual monographs prepared by experts in the fields of clinical child psychology, child psychiatry, child development, and related disciplines. The primary focus is on developmental psychopathology, which refers broadly here to the diagnosis, assessment, treatment, and prevention of problems that arise in the period from infancy through adolescence. A working assumption of the series is that understanding, identifying, and

vii

treating problems of youth must draw on multiple disciplines and diverse views within a given discipline.

The task for individual contributors is to present the latest theory and research on various topics, including specific types of dysfunction, diagnostic and treatment approaches, and special problem areas that affect adjustment. Core topics within clinical work are addressed by the series. Authors are asked to bridge potential theory, research, and clinical practice and to outline the current status and future directions. The goals of the series and the tasks presented to individual contributors are demanding. We have been extremely fortunate in recruiting leaders in the fields who have been able to translate their recognized scholarship and expertise into highly readable works on contemporary topics.

The topic of adolescent pregnancy and childbearing is broad in scope because it at once entails multiple issues related to sexual activity, development, and parenting, each with its own sweeping consequence. In the present book, Laurie Schwab Zabin and Sarah C. Hayward provide an integrative approach to the topic and issues by weaving empirical research from diverse perspectives related to adolescent pregnancy. Biological, sociocultural, and interpersonal forces and influences impinging on adolescents are discussed, all within a developmental framework. Among the topics, patterns of sexual activity, contraceptive use, abortion, single parenthood, adolescent relationships, prenatal care, and interventions to prevent adolescent pregnancy are accorded major attention. Many of the topics are laden with value issues and social concerns. The very special expertise of the authors, their own programmatic research in this area, and their unusual ability to integrate current findings from several areas yield a pivotal statement of the issues for research and social policy.

—*Alan E. Kazdin, Ph.D.*

PREFACE

Any author is likely to see his or her field of exploration as infinitely complex, perhaps because the woods begin to disappear in the trees, or perhaps because looking at any subject too long tends to multiply and magnify the issues. The social, economic, medical, and moral implications of adolescent sexual behavior and childbearing suggest many potential approaches to the field and also result in a vast and growing literature from each of these disciplinary perspectives. And the political implications of any perspective on adolescent pregnancy can only add to problems of its definition or explanation, as indeed they tend to confuse issues of prevention and management.

We have attempted to draw from a large literature in our discussions, but we do not pretend to approach all aspects of the subject without opinions and value judgments. We address the demography of adolescent pregnancy, the etiology of sexual onset, the management of sexual relationships and childbearing, and to some extent, intervention. Although we have not masked our point of view, we have tried to suggest the areas in which there is debate and to clarify the dimensions of those debates even when we only touch on them here. It should be clear when we are reporting the objective findings of research in the field—including our own—and when we are proposing a particular vision of the problem and what we hope are directions for its amelioration. Our belief that adolescents are basically rational beings and that the problem—to the extent that it is objectively a problem—is rooted deeply in our society and in the major social and economic dilemmas of our time is shared by many scholars in the field. We hope we have not suggested that it is totally amenable to categoric intervention on the one hand or that it is totally dependent on major social change on the other. Somewhere in between may give us a little—but not too much—hope.

Many funders have supported our research over the last years, research on which this book draws heavily. Credit should be given in particular to the Ford Foundation, whose core support has not only funded much of the research but also has provided a modicum of time to report on it. Thanks are due as well to the many colleagues who have been part of our research endeavors and especially to Janet B. Hardy, M.D.C.M.; it was in hammering out our joint work on *Adolescent Pregnancy in an Urban Environment* (Hardy & Zabin, 1991) that many of the ideas discussed here were refined. The superb students who take my course in adolescent pregnancy have contributed more than they know—their insights, challenges, and discussions introduce new ideas and new perspectives year after year. We still have much to learn.

—*Laurie Schwab Zabin, Ph.D.*

1

INTRODUCTION

Childbearing in adolescence is not an isolated event. It is the end point of a series of behaviors that begins with the onset of sexual activity and continues through coitus, contraception, conception, and pregnancy to either abortion or childbearing. Each behavior requires a decision, conscious or unconscious; as with all fertility issues, these decisions are infinitely complex in their consequences. Reproductive decisions, whether among adolescents or adults, affect all dimensions of human life, from the individual, the couple, and the family, to the community, the nation, and the world. And, as personal as these decisions may appear to be, fertility and its management have social implications that touch realms as diverse as medicine and ethics, science and religion, psychology and economics, and unfortunately even politics. The complexity of the demographic issues implicit in each of these areas is probably matched only by the strength of the opinions and emotions they evoke. This is never more true than in the case of adolescent pregnancy.

An individual adolescent's decisions about sexuality and fertility are constrained by the customs and sanctions of a particular cultural group. Nevertheless all cultural groups in the United States appear to regard a similar pattern for the life course as optimal. Whether for moral, economic, or social reasons, the normative life schedule is to complete schooling, gain employment, get married, and then undertake parenthood. Although families in most socioeconomic, ethnic, and cultural settings will voice that norm and aspire to it, the strength of this ordering varies according to the perceived rewards of conforming to it and the perceived penalties of diverging from it.

In most societies, out-of-wedlock pregnancy and childbearing in adolescence violate this optimal pattern. Although they often result in a personal, as well as a very real, social dilemma, it must be recognized from the outset that it is not the behaviors themselves that are problematic, but

1

their timing. It is primarily age that makes the adolescent transition to coital activity and conception problematic. Childbearing and the desire to experience sexual contact are biologically normal once physical maturation has occurred. For this reason, premature sexual activity is unlike the socially unacceptable behaviors with which it is often grouped. Illicit drug use, alcohol abuse, and delinquency are damaging at whatever age they occur and are never considered normative by the society at large. It is the age at which early sexual onset and pregnancy occur that, by placing them generally outside marriage and interfering with what is perceived as a normative progression of life events, defines them as "problem" or "high-risk" behaviors.

Moreover, the age at which an adolescent becomes a parent will in large part determine the severity of the disruption he or she will experience. Such an interruption of the tasks of adolescent development, truncating as it often does the completion of schooling and the opportunity to build a strong, independent life, contributes to the individual and social implications of premature parenting. The issue of age therefore must be central to any analysis of adolescent conception.

The Implications of Age

Although the term *teen pregnancy* has captured popular attention, it cannot capture the complexity of youthful fertility behavior. Those who understand adolescence are aware of the importance of more subtle age distinctions than the word *teenager* implies. Adolescence is preeminently a period of flux, of change, and of growth; there is no period, with the possible exception of infancy, in which age plays so important and complex a part. The role of chronological age, however, is particularly confusing because the stages of adolescence are timed differently for each individual. Physical, emotional, moral, and mental development appear to follow well-described sequences that are similar from one individual to another, but even within one individual, each proceeds on a different track. The timetables observed by these areas of development are often different; they are rarely in synchrony. If these discontinuities make it dangerous to generalize about youthful sexual behavior, they also compound the difficulty of designing appropriate interventions. And they make it difficult to muster the societal support that is required to address adolescent sexual, contraceptive, and fertility behavior, and thus they complicate issues of public policy that plague the field. This is because a programmatic response that is acceptable to the community for one age group may not appear acceptable for another, even when both groups are demonstrably at risk.

Although many of the differences in sexual activity and pregnancy among younger and older teens are matters of degree, some are actually differences of kind. Sex and pregnancy in later adolescence probably have been affected by the same societal changes that have had their impact on adult out-of-wedlock or extramarital behavior. The "revolution" that occurred over the last 20 years in the sexual behavior of younger and older adults has inevitably filtered down to the teenage population. Messages communicated by the media and patterns of behavior observed among their older peers have changed teenagers' sexual norms in virtually all areas of the country in ways that have cut across ethnic, religious, and social groups. In early adolescence, however, we are looking at a rather different phenomenon.

Sex play immediately following puberty—or even preceding it—and early postpubertal conception appear to have different characteristics and more severe consequences than those same behaviors might have a few years later. Their etiology is clearly different. And, rather than being characteristic of all geographic settings, very early coital behaviors are generally much more common among disadvantaged young people. These behaviors typically cluster in deprived urban communities where other high-risk activities target poor, often minority, neighborhoods. Whereas sexually transmitted diseases, unintended pregnancy, and abortion result from sexual activity in older and younger teen populations alike, in any social or economic group, premarital childbearing is a more frequent outcome among poor, economically isolated populations.

Why do the consequences of teenage sexual activity tend to differ with age? Older teenagers of 18 or 19 years will in general have ceased growing. Those who delay sexual onset until their later teens will be more mature in their cognitive and socioemotional development. Many will have finished high school, some will be working, and some will be married. Their obstetrical risks, if they conceive, will on average be lower than those of younger teenagers (unless they have already borne a child during their early adolescence, in which case their risks will be increased). Although their social risks will in general be higher than those of women who delay their first birth until 20 years or older, especially if the teenager is a single parent living in a disadvantaged environment, they usually will be lower than those of younger teens.

Pregnant adolescents younger than age 18, on the other hand, are usually at high risk both medically and socially. They are generally still growing and therefore may be in competition with the fetus for nutrients. The likelihood of anemia, which is common during the normal adolescent growth spurt, is increased by pregnancy, and other complications of pregnancy are frequent. As a result, in the absence of comprehensive and specialized prenatal care, preterm delivery and low infant birth weight occur with higher frequency in this age group than in women who commence childbearing later. Premature termination of schooling, single parenthood, repeated and unintended pregnancy, difficulties in obtaining employment, and economic dependency are commonplace among mothers who start childbearing as adolescents. Therefore the costs borne by the offspring and families of adolescent mothers, as well as by the young mothers themselves, are often higher than those experienced by those who first bear children in the later teen years. And after the child is born, personal characteristics of the young mother that are normal during her own adolescent development are often the antithesis of those attributes required for successful parenting.

Legal as well as developmental issues separate adolescents of 17 years and younger from older teenagers. In most states, the age of majority is 18 years; adolescents are minors, in most instances still dependent on parents for physical, psychosocial, and financial support. Older teenagers are, at least in legal terms, independent and able to make decisions on their own. Fortunately, laws in many states allow minors to make confidential reproductive health decisions; the professionals to whom they turn are expected to grant them that right. Nonetheless, the distinction between minors and older teenagers is a common one; despite the legal requirement that they serve adolescents confidentially, many clinicians feel quite differently when faced with a legally "emancipated" teenager from when they see their patient as an "adult."

There is a long-standing tradition in vital statistics that groups together ages 15-19 years when reporting pregnancies and births. This tradition has supported a broad definition of *adolescence* but for many purposes has been counterproductive. It omits the pubertal years below 15 and treats young females with markedly different developmental characteristics as if they were members of a homogenous group. Data based on that formulation can result in misleading conclusions about the effects of adolescent childbearing because, whereas 18 and 19 years of age may be optimal for childbearing from the biological point of view, some negative effects are observed even with the best of care among pregnant girls under 16 years of age.

Another definition of adolescence refers to ages 10-18, describing those years as a still-dependent period from early puberty through high school (U.S. Congress, 1991). Similarly, in the lay press, adolescence can often be understood as the loosely defined period of life that extends from puberty through the teen years to adulthood. Clearly, we need a more subtle analysis of age differences within adolescence. Only in such a context can we understand the etiology, nature, and effects of adolescent childbearing. Age works through psychosocial, economic, and biological mechanisms, differentially in different socioeconomic settings, to influence the onset of sexual behavior, the risk of conception, choices with respect to contraception and pregnancy outcome, and the sequelae of childbirth. Thus, whether we consider the causes or consequences of "teenage" pregnancy, its occurrence or its avoidance, it is a very different phenomenon when it occurs at different developmental periods during the second decade of life.

We believe that these distinctions are not merely academic; semantics may have stood in the way of society's response to this apparently intransigent social dilemma. What is seen as a matter of conscious choice in some settings and at some ages may in other settings and at other ages be understood as a product of environment and circumstance. That distinction has implications for intervention that may be lost when the issue is seen as monolithic.

Definitions

Adolescents Versus Teens. We will use a narrower definition of adolescent pregnancy as we address it in the presence of the developmental diversity of the teen years. Any definition based on chronological age is necessarily arbitrary, but we will consider adolescents those who are 17 years and younger. We will not focus on the needs of the 18- or 19-year-old young adult, although many are still dependent and living with their parents. We will focus on young people from the age of puberty, which may occur as early as 9 or 10 or as late as 15 or 16 years of age, through the age of 17. Even within that span, the characteristics of a 13-year-old child who becomes a mother are vastly different from those of a 17-year-old who is about to graduate from high school or even a 16-year-old whose schooling is interrupted by motherhood. We will consider the implications of many of those differences.

Pregnancy Versus Childbearing. Another semantic distinction should be noted at the outset: the distinction between pregnancy and childbearing. Much of the work on adolescent pregnancy has focused on the sequelae of too-early parenting. Unfortunately the term *pregnancy* is often used instead of *childbearing.* Pregnancies, however, frequently do not end with a birth, especially among adolescents. It is only in these age groups that the numbers of pregnancies terminated by abortion approach those of live births; under 15 years of age, the number of abortions actually exceeds that of births. Although a high abortion rate should, of itself, provide an impetus to preventive intervention, it must be noted that the many detrimental consequences of adolescent pregnancy reported in the literature do not occur when a pregnancy is terminated with induced abortion. It has been shown that abortion is a safe medical procedure for this age group, safer at all gestational periods than childbirth (Cates, Schultz, & Grimes, 1983; Grimes & Cates, 1979). More recently, there is evidence that it has virtually no negative psychological sequelae and that the young women who choose this option bear none of the negative economic and educational consequences that plague so many young mothers (Zabin, Hirsch, & Emerson, 1989). They are less likely to have another unintended conception in the period subsequent to that outcome than are those who carry to term. It is essential, therefore, to consider pregnancy and childbearing separately and to make explicit that distinction.

The Two Problems of Teenage Pregnancy

We would suggest that there are at least two problems of teenage pregnancy. One relates to those young people who initiate intercourse in their late teenage years. In general, they are more likely to use contraception and to avoid childbearing until after their schooling is complete. The other relates to those frequently disadvantaged young women whose sexual onset is during their pubertal years, whose pregnancies are likely to be premature, and whose conceptions are more likely to result in childbearing. There are legal and policy implications of those distinctions, just as there are developmental and clinical reasons for regarding age as a salient factor in an analysis of the problem. This recognition suggests that many of the interventions that are likely to help older teenagers avoid pregnancy may be insufficient by themselves to help those who are at risk of conceiving during their adolescent years.

The Pages That Follow

In the next chapter, we will summarize data on recent trends in the several components of adolescent fertility and its social context. We then will discuss sexual onset and the many developmental and normative influences on it. We will explore adolescent sexual and contraceptive behaviors and the characteristics of adolescents that shape their conduct. We will discuss the etiology and consequences of childbearing and the effects of optimal prenatal care. And we will present a range of interventions that have been essayed and will discuss the roles that professionals in many disciplines can play in helping young people manage their sexual and reproductive lives. At each stage, we will attempt to see the adolescent as a product of the intergenerational and social forces that impinge on him or her.

It is difficult to remember, particularly when we focus on young adolescents, that another generation is already in the making. The same influences that are affecting their youthful behaviors are now or soon will be the parental influences they pass on to their children. There is very little time to intervene.

2

ADOLESCENT PREGNANCY IN THE UNITED STATES

INTRODUCTION

When adolescent pregnancy is described as an epidemic, the term is misleading. It implies not only that adolescent conceptions affect large segments of the population but also that they have arisen spontaneously at some moment in time and can be expected to disappear spontaneously—or when we learn how to deal with them effectively. In fact, early conception and childbearing are not sudden or passing phenomena. They have deep roots in the past and will have ramifications for years to come.

The United States has a long history of relatively early childbearing, albeit in the context of early marriage. Rates of premarital pregnancy have undergone cyclical variations over the last three centuries, with peaks in the late 18th century and in recent years (Smith, 1978). Historical changes in recent decades, however, have profoundly altered the societal context within which adolescent sexual behavior occurs. During the 1960s and 1970s, the social, economic, and cultural context of adolescence changed (Hayes, 1987). Within this altered social context, adolescent pregnancy and childbearing were given new parameters and their occurrences became more visible, although they were not necessarily more common. The social change that led to this visibility appears profound and rapid, but in many ways it constitutes a change in the nature of adolescence as much as it is a change in fertility behaviors themselves.

THE EMERGENCE OF THE
ADOLESCENT PREGNANCY ISSUE

What are some of those changes? The average age at menarche has declined; the average age at marriage has risen, and marriage patterns are less homogenous; economic shifts have led simultaneously to a need for longer educational careers and to pockets of intractable urban poverty where education is often truncated. Concurrently, sexual norms across society have altered. These trends have had an effect on the length and the quality of the teenage years and more specifically on the nature and risks of the transition to adulthood which we call adolescence. Their effects on sexual activity and childbearing are discussed below.

In comparison to the transitions evident in the 19th century, while the transitions that characterize participation in today's adult world—exit from school, entrance into the work force, departure from the family of origin, marriage and establishment of a household—have become more concentrated and more universal, they are generally initiated later (Modell, Furstenberg, & Hershberg, 1978). Their sequencing has become more complex as the conflicting demands of each transition coincide one with the other. Thus young people must wait longer to begin the shift to adulthood but face more complex decisions when they do. Deviations from this rigid but later normative timing have become more aberrant and costly.

Maturation and Marriage

Adolescence itself is, of course, a socially defined period, insofar as a particular culture acknowledges such a period at all. As long as a culture limits male-female contact to socially prescribed interactions from puberty to marriage, as long as legitimated unions take place at a time relatively close to physical maturation, or as long as strict regulations govern behaviors during that interval, adolescent pregnancy is not an important issue, nor, if the interval is brief, is adolescence itself. In the Western world at the present time, however, intervals between physical maturation and legitimated union are often very long. The age of physical maturation among females in the Western world has been declining and is currently stabilized at a mean menarcheal age of approximately 12.5 years (see Chapter 3). Problems of pregnancy understandably can become acute in nations where menarche is occurring earlier, making it possible to conceive at much younger ages. While the age of physical maturation has shifted downward, the normative age of marriage, for various reasons, has shifted upward. These reasons encompass the changing roles of women, their participation in the labor force, the cost of maintaining a conjugal home, the increased role of cohabitation both as a precursor to marriage and independent of marriage, the cost of childrearing, and the growing importance of a prolonged education. The proportion of teenagers who are married declined throughout the 1960s and 1970s (Hayes, 1987). In 1960, 84% of females and 96% of males under age 20 were single, but by 1984 these proportions had risen to 93% and 98.5%, respectively. During this same interval, the median age at first marriage rose from slightly over age 20 to almost 23 for women and from almost age 23 to over 25 for men (Bureau of the Census, 1984). The sharpest decrease in rates of marriage occurred among blacks: The percentage of black female 15- to 19-year-olds ever-married dropped from 16.2% in 1960 to 1.6% in 1984, while for males the change was from 3.4% to 1.8% (Hayes, 1987). The only ethnic group in which teenage marriage became more likely was the Hispanic population, which has higher rates of marriage among teenagers than either the black or white population. The lower likelihood of marrying affected primarily older teenagers, of 18 and 19 years. Teenagers of 15-17 years have always had very low rates of marriage, but in this age group, 7% were married in 1960 and only 2% in 1984 (Hayes, 1987). Such changes in marriage patterns have brought concomitant increases in single parenthood and absentee fathering, with pronounced social and economic consequences.

Education and Employment

The economic system into which young people are absorbed has required a longer educational incubation at a time when inequalities in access to economic and educational opportunities have widened and in fact have been exacerbated by economic changes. Although the percentage of teenagers enrolled in school has remained constant for about two decades at 98% of 14- to 15-year-olds, 92% of 16- to 17-year-olds, and 50% of 18- to 19-year-olds, (Bureau of the Census, 1985; Hayes, 1987) the rate of school attendance in high-risk populations is lower, and the impact of a poor educational preparation is more severe (Modell, 1989). The configuration of the labor force has changed; the market for unskilled labor has contracted. The need for higher education is reflected in the fact that only at levels *after* high school has enrollment increased in recent years, and only in the late teens are whites more likely than blacks to enroll in an educational institution (Hayes, 1987). Although high rates of school enrollment exist nationally, working during the school years is also common, with 6.3 million teenagers employed part- or full-time. However, this economic role is not equally available to all subgroups: 48% of white 16- to 19-year-olds were employed in 1985, compared with 25% of blacks in that age group. The unemployment statistics also reflect the difficulty some groups experience in entering the work force: 41% of black teenagers over age 16 were registered as unemployed in 1985, compared with 16% of whites (Hayes, 1987). In fact, the employment rate among school-enrolled teenagers has been rising since World War II, while that among teenagers out of school has been decreasing (Modell, 1989). Thus the demands of the economy and the availability of education have extended the period of dependence for most young people in comparison with that of 20 or 30 years ago and have left some groups without access to the economic options that encourage them to prepare for the future.

The Sexual Revolution

Many aspects of sexual and fertility behavior were altering during this period, including the norms surrounding premarital intercourse. Rates of sexual initiation among adolescents rose dramatically through the 1970s, with higher percentages of teenagers experiencing coitus at younger and younger ages (Zelnik & Kantner, 1980). In large measure, these behaviors reflected changes that also occurred among young adults and older women, but whereas some of those changes were observed throughout the country, very early sexual initiation and childbearing were concentrated among the disadvantaged. One might speculate that some of the pressure for change resulted indirectly from younger ages at physical maturation. Although changes in sexual behavior and changes in physical maturation did not occur simultaneously, it is reasonable to propose that biological pressures could have had their social impact a generation or two later, when they coincided with other dramatic changes in sexual behavior and the role of women. Adolescent sexual onset and childbearing may have become more or less common in proportion to the strength of the rewards society offers for resisting those pressures; where rewards are few, one would expect that social restraints would be less powerful—an interpretation of sexual onset that we will address more fully below.

Thus adolescence became a longer and more complex period of life, and sexuality outside marriage gained in acceptance. At the time of these changes, the large group of "baby boomers" were reaching their teens. The U.S. population between the ages of 13 and 19 peaked in

1976 at 21.4 million (Hayes, 1987). In the 1980s, it declined, reaching an estimated 16.9 million in 1990 (Bureau of the Census, 1986) but it will increase again as the children of the baby boom generation reach adolescence. The surge in the numbers of teenagers during the late 1960s and 1970s meant that anything teenagers were doing tended to command attention. And what they were doing was often quite different from what their parents had done. On the average, they were marrying later and engaging in sex earlier.

Demographic trends such as these do not occur in a vacuum. Legal reforms also occurred that increased the visibility of adolescent conceptions. Abortions were legalized in 1973, and from 1975 on, Title IX of the 1972 Education Act made it illegal for schools to require pregnant girls to leave. During the 1960s and 1970s, the last legal barriers to contraceptive use came down. Although they had not stood in the way of contraceptive distribution to most citizens in most parts of the country, that signalled an important change in availability of contraception to those who depended on public support: The first federal funding for family planning clinics began in the mid-1960s, and distribution networks grew through the 1970s. In that context, adolescent pregnancy became more visible as the ability of older women to prevent unwanted childbearing improved. With the increased availability of effective methods of contraception, differentials between adult economic and racial subgroups diminished in their rates of unintended pregnancy; adolescents stood out as one of the last remaining groups who were unable to control their fertility. During this period, the media acquired more power to reach young people and treated sexual matters in increasingly explicit ways. It has never been demonstrated that watching television promotes sexual activity, but it seems clear that changes in the treatment of sexual behavior reflected changes in the level of permissiveness across the country as a whole.

The changes that occurred, particularly during the 1970s, were remarkable in their magnitude and rapidity. Cultural patterns that circumscribe the formation of unions between men and women and thus affect the context of human reproduction often remain constant for generations. In one decade, however, measurable change occurred. Public pronouncements on the subject of adolescent pregnancy became vociferous, not only as a result of that rapidity of change but also as this concern became entwined in the moral, legal, and political debates through which attitudes toward other societal changes were expressed.

Values regarding the nature of the family and its structure, opinions about the obligations of society with regard to sexuality and childbearing, and attitudes toward the roles of men and women are all undercurrents in this debate—sometimes tacit, sometimes not. Within this context, it is not surprising to find that the "problem" of adolescent conception, impelled by differing value systems, can be very differently defined. From one perspective, sexual intercourse may be seen as the problem, while from another, it is only when babies are born to adolescent mothers that their behavior becomes a matter of societal concern. From another perspective, abortion is the primary issue; from yet another, sexually transmitted diseases, including AIDS. Each of these emphases has contributed to the emergence of adolescent pregnancy on the social agenda; each suggests an appropriate but different point of intervention. All must command our attention.

ADOLESCENT FERTILITY BEHAVIORS

Because adolescent childbearing is a composite outcome of numerous social and demographic processes, the statistics describing it have to be used with care, separating each of the underlying phenomena that enter into an adolescent fertility rate. Changes in the rates of one component of fertility may relate to the overall fertility rate in ways that are not intuitively apparent, because two components of fertility—frequency of coitus and frequency of conception, for example—may be moving in opposite directions (Hayes, 1987). If all the components in the demographic picture are not accurately assessed, program and policy decisions can miss the mark and may even be counterproductive.

The birth rate among all teenagers, for example, depends on three underlying behaviors: sexual activity, the use of contraception, and recourse to abortion after conception. The birth rate among the sexually active alone depends on the use and effectiveness of contraception and on the abortion/childbirth ratio. As we shall see, the pregnancy rate in the teenage population as a whole may be rising while the birth rate is declining. The pregnancy rate among sexually active teenagers may be declining, while among all teenagers, it is rising. Contraceptive practices may be improving even though abortion rates may be increasing. Aggregate figures that summarize these rates can be understood only in the context of the larger demographic picture.

The Size of the Adolescent Population

One central influence on perceptions of adolescent pregnancy and birth is the relative size of the teenage population. Fluctuations in the numbers and proportion of teenagers in the population have an impact not only on the total numbers of births to the age group but also on the proportion of all births contributed by them. Even within the teenage population, individual age cohorts can influence the statistics. If there is a rapidly rising teenage population, there will be an increase in the proportion of younger teens, whereas in a declining teenage population, there will be more older teens. Given higher birth and pregnancy rates at the older ages, the rates for the 15- to 19-year-old population as a whole are affected by the age balance within it. As noted above, the teenage population has been decreasing since 1976, and the number of pregnancies and births to this age group also has been decreasing.

Not only is the size of the teenage population as a whole changing, but its composition also changes with time. Minorities constitute an increasing percentage of teenagers, with black youth making up 14% of this population and Hispanics 7% in 1984 (Hayes, 1987). As these proportions rise, the distribution of subgroups across the nation is also shifting; in some urban areas they are and/or will be in the majority, and, to the extent that their fertility rates differ from those of the white majority, the overall level of teenage childbearing will be affected.

Births to Teenagers

The number of births to 15- to 19-year-olds has been decreasing nationwide since the early 1970s. The proportion of all U.S. births which are accounted for by teenage mothers has also declined, slowly, in the 1980s (Moore, Wenk, Hofferth, & Hayes, 1987). In large part, these trends are due to a shrinking teenage population, a declining teenage birth rate, and an increase in births overall as the baby boom generation reached its 30s.

In 1972, there were 616,280 births to women 15-19 years old (Moore, Wenk, Hofferth & Hayes, 1987), whereas in 1988, there were 488,941 to women under 20 years old, with 10,558 to girls younger than 15 years (Alan Guttmacher Institute [AGI], 1991). As a proportion of all births, those to teenagers 15-19 years old declined from 19% in 1972 to 12% in 1986 (Moore et al., 1987). When only first births are considered, however, 23% of first-time mothers in 1988 were teenagers (AGI, 1991). Approximately 73% of births to teenagers in 1988 were unintended, up from 67%

in 1982; 80% of these unintended births occurred sooner than the mothers had wanted, the remaining 20% were to mothers who did not want a child at any time (Forrest & Singh, 1990).

The birth rate to teenagers as a whole declined from the early 1970s to the mid-1980s (Moore et al., 1987) but rose slightly between 1984 and 1988. In 1972, there were 65 births per 1,000 15- to 19-year-old females; in 1984, 51 births per 1,000; and in 1988, 53.6 per 1,000 (AGI, 1991). The birth rate among 15- to 17-year-olds rose 10% between 1986 and 1988 to its highest level since 1977 (AGI, 1991).

The demographic impact of births to teenagers, and specifically to young teenagers, varies by ethnic group. Compared with the national average of 12%, nearly 23% of births among the black population and 19% among native Americans are to teenagers (National Center for Health Statistics, 1988). Overall, of births to women under age 20, 38% are to mothers 17 years of age or younger; but among black Americans, this figure is 45.4%. These discrepancies suggest the impact of environmental, economic, and cultural conditions on the risk of adolescent conception and birth.

Pregnancies Among Teenagers

Despite declining birth rates, rates of pregnancy among teenagers have increased. The likelihood that a teenage girl will experience a pregnancy steadily increased from 1972 to 1980 as the pregnancy rate among 15- to 19-year-old females rose from 94 to 111 per 1,000. The pregnancy rate stabilized in the 1980s; it has been 109 per 1,000 since 1984 (AGI, 1991). To some extent, the discrepancy between pregnancy and birth rate trends reflects increased recourse to abortion to prevent an unwanted birth. The pregnancy rates, on the other hand, do not reflect less effective contraceptive practices. On the contrary, when only *sexually active* teenagers are considered, their pregnancy rate declined from 272 per 1,000 in 1972 to 243 per 1,000 in 1987; because these changes accelerated over time, they included a drop of 10% in the last 5 years alone (Forrest & Singh, 1990), all of which was attributable to improved levels of contraceptive use (Hayes, 1987).

In all, more than 1 million pregnancies occur among teenagers each year in the United States (AGI, 1991). Studies repeatedly indicate that more than 80% of these pregnancies—90% among unmarried teenagers— are unintended (AGI, 1991; Forrest & Singh, 1990; Zelnik & Kantner, 1980). In fact, rates of unintended pregnancy have risen, while overall pregnancy rates have fallen (Forrest & Singh, 1990). Not surprisingly, therefore, only half of these pregnancies result in a live birth; an estimated 36% terminate with an elective abortion, and approximately 14% result in miscarriage (AGI, 1991). It has been estimated that 40% of white and 63% of black 15- to 19-year-olds experience a first pregnancy under age 20; 21% and 40%, respectively, will do so by age 18 (Forrest, 1986). Minority teenagers are at more than twice the risk of whites.

Sexual Activity Among Teenagers

Rates of sexual activity and contraceptive use explain these trends; that is, they explain why there has been a rise in pregnancy rates among all teenagers while pregnancies decline among those who are sexually active. *Sexually active* by convention has meant "having experienced intercourse at least once." This definition is a very narrow yardstick of sexual activity and pregnancy risk; it does not take into account the frequency of intercourse, numbers of partners, or many other telling factors that are central to judgments about an individual's level of sexual contact. Nor does it reflect differences between the behaviors of groups or individuals at any one point in time, nor differences over time in the behavior of a single individual or group. Nevertheless it is an indicator that can be assessed with relative ease, and research has relied heavily on it.

Prior to the 1970s, there were few data about sexual activity among the population as a whole or among teenagers. Most of what was known came from nonprobability surveys conducted by Kinsey et al. (Kinsey, Pomeroy, & Martin, 1948; Kinsey, Pomeroy, Martin, & Gebhard, 1953) who estimated that in the years between 1938 and 1950, 7% of white females had experienced intercourse by age 16. The landmark studies of Zelnik and Kantner (1973, 1977, 1980) and Zelnik & Shah (1983) charted a remarkable change in the behavior of teenagers. In 1971, 27.6% of never-married females aged 15-19 had experienced intercourse; in 1979, that proportion was 46.0%. Between those years, there was a 50% increase in the percentage of 15-year-old girls who had experienced coitus; in 1972, 14.4% had had intercourse at this age, whereas in 1979, 22.5% had done so. Overall, 50% of 15- to 19-year-olds in metropolitan areas were sexually active in 1979, compared with 30% in 1971.

In the early 1980s, rates of sexual activity among teenagers appeared to stabilize and even drop, to 42.2% in 1982 (Hayes, 1987; Hofferth &

Hayes, 1987). However, recent data from the 1988 National Survey of Family Growth indicate that rates have continued to rise during the last decade, with 49.5% of never-married females aged 15-19 having experienced intercourse; among all women of this age, 53% are now sexually active (Forrest & Singh, 1990). Thus more than half of 15- to 19-year-old women have initiated sexual activity. Furthermore, the trend toward stabilization does not appear in the youngest groups (Hofferth, Kahn, & Baldwin, 1987). Although the trend toward more coital activity appeared to peak among older teens, more and more young people of 16 years and below are still becoming sexually active and at younger ages.

Young men have consistently reported earlier sexual experience than young women. Among never-married males aged 15 to 19, three out of five reported that they have had sexual intercourse. This proportion translates into a cumulative percentage of 80% of young men having had intercourse by the time they are 20 years old (Sonenstein, Pleck, & Ku, 1991). Among women, 75% of 18- to 19-year-olds have experienced coitus (Forrest & Singh, 1990), but at younger ages the differential between males and females is more pronounced. For example, in 1983, 16.6% of males had experienced intercourse by age 15, compared with 5.4% of females; by age 17, 48% of males and 27% of females were sexually active; and by age 19, the rates were 78% and 63%, respectively (Hayes, 1987). As more young people become sexually active, males and females alike are experiencing coitus at younger and younger ages; these ages are especially low among males. The mean age of coital contact for females who start in their teens is 16.2 years; among males, it is 15.7 years (AGI, 1991). Two out of five males are sexually active at 15 years, eight out of ten by 19 years; one out of four females is sexually active by 15 years, seven out of ten by 19 years.

In addition to gender differentials, rates of sexual activity vary by race and ethnicity, although these differences have been declining over the past two decades. In 1971, the proportion of black teenagers who were sexually active was 30% higher than that among white teenagers (Zelnik & Kantner, 1980). By 1982, that difference was only 13% (Hayes, 1987), and it has continued to narrow. Among women in 1982, non-Hispanic white teenagers had the lowest level of sexual activity, 15 percentage points lower than that of non-Hispanic blacks; by 1988, the differential had narrowed to only 8 percentage points (Forrest & Singh, 1990). The gender disparity in rates of sexual activity has also decreased, although it remains larger within the black population. Averages tend to mask extremes: In an urban, black population, the average age of first intercourse was reported as 12 by males and 14 by females (Zabin, Smith, Hirsch, & Hardy, 1986). These data are consistent with younger ages of sexual onset in the black population on average (Zelnik & Shah, 1983). Gender and racial differences are greatest in the early teens and decline with age (Hayes, 1987). It is important to note that race, in this case, is in large measure a proxy for social and economic disadvantage; rates of sexual activity have been shown to be negatively related to socioeconomic status and schooling, a relationship that holds among all racial groups. Recent increases in rates of sexual activity among young women, however, have occurred almost entirely in the white, nonpoor population and have thereby narrowed socioeconomic differentials as well (Forrest & Singh, 1990).

Contraceptive Use

The use of contraception can be measured in a number of ways. Whether contraception has ever or never been used in any coital act is one way; researchers also refer to a specific coital occasion, such as first intercourse, as a measure of preparedness for sexual onset, or last intercourse, which, viewed as a random event, gives some estimate of consistency of use. Histories, or time-trend studies, are complex to elicit and analyze, due to differences in measures, methods, and definitions of effective use.

The use of contraception at first intercourse by American women rose dramatically in the 1980s. Between 1965 and 1979, the proportion using a method remained stable, at about 44% to 47%. In the early 1980s, this proportion increased to 53%, and to 65% between 1983 and 1988 (Mosher & McNally, 1991). The increase was attributable to the increasing use of condoms during the 1980s. In 1975-1979, 22% of women stated that at first intercourse their partner had used a condom, whereas in 1983-1988, this figure was 42%. The proportion of women who used other methods has remained essentially the same since 1965, except for a small increase in pill use between the late 1960s and early 1970s (Mosher & McNally, 1991). Throughout this period, the condom has been the most common method of contraception at first coitus but, nonetheless, one in three women remains unprotected at this event (AGI, 1991).

In 1988, 79% of sexually active 15- to 19-year-old women indicated that they used contraception, an increase from 71% in 1982. Nevertheless, teenagers remain more likely than other age groups to use no method, with one in five being a nonuser (AGI, 1991). Poor women exposed to unintended pregnancy are much more likely not to be using a contraceptive method, and among poor teenagers this proportion reaches 25% (Forrest & Singh, 1990).

The most recent data about male adolescent sexual behavior corroborates the conclusion that condom use increased substantially in the 1980s. In 1988, condom use among sexually active metropolitan 17- to 19-year-old males had more than doubled, with 58% reporting that they had used a condom the last time they had intercourse, compared with 21% in 1979 (Sonenstein, Pleck, & Ku, 1989). At *first* intercourse, 55% of young men said that they had used a condom, compared with a low 7% or 9% use of effective female methods in 1988 and 1979, respectively. At *last* intercourse, the use of effective female methods without condoms decreased slightly; in 1988, 22% of young men reported such use, compared with 28% in 1979. But the proportion using ineffective contraception or no method at last coitus dropped from over 50% to 23% (Sonenstein et al., 1989).

Racial and ethnic differences in contraceptive use are in evidence. The increase in condom use is dramatic in all groups but is greatest among black males: The proportion using a condom at *last* intercourse rose from 23% to 62% between 1979 and 1988, compared with a rise from 21% to 57% among nonblacks. At *first* coitus, however, blacks are less likely to use a condom and more likely to use no protection, probably as a result of their earlier ages of coital onset (Sonenstein et al., 1989).

In all, contraceptive practices among teenagers have improved over the last two decades: The condom has become a more important method at first intercourse and at all ages. Young men and young women report increased reliance on this method. Because the use of female methods has dropped only slightly, condom use generally has replaced nonuse rather than replacing medical contraception.

Abortion

Although abortion rates increased after legalization in 1973, the abortion rate among teenagers has been essentially stable since the late 1970s. Four in ten teenage pregnancies (excluding miscarriages) end in abortion. In 1987, there were approximately 406,790 abortions to women under age 20 (AGI, 1991), and the estimate for 1977 was not significantly different (Tietze, 1978). The under-20 age group accounts for 26% of all abortions in the United States each year. The teenage abortion rate (calculated as the number of abortions per 1,000 women aged 15-19) is twice as high among minorities as among whites. This is due to higher rates of sexual activity, lower rates of contraceptive use, and thus more unintended pregnancies. It does not imply a greater likelihood that minority teenagers will terminate any given pregnancy (Hayes, 1987): Their abortion ratio, describing the proportion of pregnancies that end in abortion, is no greater.

Only at the youngest ages, under 15, does the number of abortions exceed the number of live births (Hayes, 1987). High rates of unintended pregnancy among the young result each year in 4% of 15- to 19-year-old women experiencing an abortion (AGI, 1991). The proportion of all pregnancies that are terminated by abortion is twice as high among teenage women as among women aged 25-34 (Forrest & Singh, 1990). This difference results from the high level of unintended pregnancy among young women: The likelihood of ending an *unintended* pregnancy by abortion is similar at all ages up to 40 years (Forrest & Singh, 1990).

Summary of National Data

In summary, while the number of births to teenagers and the proportion of all births for which they accounted were declining in the 1970s, rates of sexual activity rose, and therefore pregnancy rates among all teenagers also rose. The age of sexual onset declined in all sectors of the population during the 1970s, and rates of sexual activity among those under age 20 continued to rise in the last decade. Disparities between the sexes and between the races are lower now than at any previous time, because recent increases have occurred primarily in the white, nonpoor population.

Contraception has contributed to a decline in the pregnancy rate among sexually active teenagers. Condom use has increased substantially in the 1980s and accounts for increased rates of contraceptive use at first and last intercourse for both men and women. The condom continues to be the most important form of contraception at first intercourse.

THE SOCIAL ENVIRONMENT

High-Risk Populations

Although nationwide statistics indicate a serious problem with premature and unwanted conception among adolescents, these figures understate the problem in high-risk populations. By combining all 15- to 19-year-olds, ignoring younger adolescents, and taking no account of the geographic distribution of the problem, adolescent conception is not represented as the severe social concern it is in poor, overcrowded, socially deprived, inner-city areas.

Hardy and Zabin (1991) reported on studies of the problem in a poor urban environment. In Baltimore, the proportion of all births accounted for by births to teenagers is 26%, more than twice the national proportion. In that city, 22% of all births are to teens. Of those births, the proportion to young teens is also much higher than nationally: over 45% of all teenage births are to mothers under age 18, with 13% to girls under age 15 who account for fewer than 5% on the national scene. Moreover the percentage of conceptions that are unintended among adolescents is higher than national estimates.

Trends in poor urban centers are not encouraging. The pregnancy rate for 14- to 17-year-olds in Baltimore continued to rise in the 1980s; although the birth rate for older teenagers may have declined somewhat in recent years, for the youngest adolescent group it has not. This indicates the importance of cohort analysis if trends are to be understood and appropriate interventions are to be designed. In poor areas, where rates are high among adolescents, the proportion of young people is growing even while it decreases for the population as a whole. This suggests the magnitude of the need for appropriate services now and in the future.

Single Parenthood

As marriage rates dropped and premarital sex became more common, the risk of premarital pregnancy almost doubled (Zelnik, Kim, & Kantner, 1979). In 1986, of all women who were under age 20 at the time of delivery, 39% were married, a figure that hides wide disparities between subgroups of the populations: 52% of white mothers under age 20 but only 10% of black mothers of this age were married. Rates of marriage at conception and delivery dropped dramatically from the 1960s to the 1980s. In the mid-1960s, about half of white teenage parents were married at the time of conception, and 85% were married by delivery; among blacks, 15% were married at conception, and 42% at delivery. In 1980, these proportions were much lower: In the white population, only 1 in 3 teenage mothers was married at conception, 2 in 3 at delivery; among black mothers, 1 in 20 was married at conception, 1 in

10 at delivery. Thus the practice of "legitimizing" a birth before delivery has become far less common.

Throughout the population, therefore, a child is more likely to be raised by a single parent than a generation ago. It is of particular concern that the younger the mother, the more likely she is to parent alone. There are estimates that in the early 1990s one in five white babies and three in four black babies will be born to single mothers (Edelman, 1988). Simultaneously there has been an increase in the proportion of women working outside the home, especially among single-parent families: 66% of single mothers with children are working, and 62% of those under age 18 are in the work force (Hayes, 1987). As suggested above, these are often the same young mothers who are attending school. Given the increased likelihood that a family headed by a single parent will live in poverty (Cherlin, 1989; Edelman, 1988), it is of concern that such families often face the multiple stresses of poverty and early parenting.

The Fathers of Babies Born to Teenagers

What do we know of the partners of young women who conceive and bear children in adolescence? Very little, compared with our knowledge of the young women themselves. In 1986, 12.6% of all women giving birth were under the age of 20, but only 2.7% of all fathers were teenagers (National Center for Health Statistics, 1988). There is a serious problem, however, with missing and scant data on paternity. Sonenstein (1986) found that, in some areas, 32% of birth records did not list the father's age; not surprisingly, this omission was especially common for out-of-wedlock births. One study showed that 2% of 18-year-old males and 4% of 19-year-old males reported being fathers, compared with 9.5% of 18-year-old and 15.5% of 19-year-old females who reported being mothers (Mott, 1983). Discrepancies with later data, however, indicate that males are not as reliable reporters of their fertility histories as females. If pregnancies end in abortion, even less is known about the male partners. These young men are rarely accessible to research or clinical intervention.

Nevertheless, in the Baltimore study, which was based on birth certificates, it was found that in 12% of all births, both parents were teenagers, while in 14%, the mother was a teenager and the father older. In only 2% of all births was the mother age 20 or older and the father a teenager. Overall, nearly 14% of all fathers were under age 20, more than fourfold the national figure of 3% (Hardy & Zabin, 1991). On the whole, fathers are older than mothers, and the age discrepancy is greater among whites than blacks. At each maternal age, white fathers are generally older than black fathers, and on average they are 4 years older than the mothers. Among black teenagers, there is on average only a 2-3 year difference between mothers' and fathers' ages.

Education

An association has been established between teenage childbearing and incomplete schooling, but the lower educational achievement of adolescent mothers is not simply a result of pregnancy. Many drop out of school *before* becoming pregnant (Upchurch & McCarthy, 1990); many others, on the basis of their prior histories, were already at risk of doing so. Nevertheless childbirth interferes with school completion, and mothers who deliver before the age of 20 have completed considerably fewer years of schooling than those who deliver between ages 20 and 24 (Hardy & Zabin, 1991). Even among those who at age 19 might have been expected to have completed high school, only 60% of white mothers and 65% of black mothers had done so (National Center for Health Statistics, 1988). Among mothers aged 17-19, more blacks than whites have finished high school, whereas among 20- to 24-year-olds, a slightly higher proportion of whites have completed 12 years of education.

The association between low educational achievement and teenage parenting also exists for young men. The Baltimore study (Hardy & Zabin, 1991) showed that among all fathers of the children parented by a teenage woman, black and white, older and younger, educational achievement was "dismal." At all ages, white fathers had fewer completed years of schooling than black fathers: Among those over 20 years old, only 28% had completed grade nine. The lower educational attainment of fathers compared with nonfathers at the same age holds for national data as well (Marsiglio, 1987).

Socioeconomic Status

Hidden beneath racial and geographic differences in all statistics in the United States lies the more serious and consistent association between adolescent conception and socioeconomic deprivation. One way to illustrate this association is to chart the geographical distribution of births and abortions to adolescents in a city. By doing this in their study of Baltimore, Hardy and Zabin (1991) found that births to those under age 18 were concentrated in the four most poverty-stricken areas of the city, both among blacks and whites. Although, with fewer numbers, the pattern among white teenagers is less intense, it nevertheless follows the same distribution. There are few births to adolescents in the affluent census tracts of the city. Abortions, although much more widely distributed than births, also are concentrated in the poorest areas. Young white mothers appear to be at greater disadvantage than young black mothers, having less education, less parental support, and poorer health for themselves and their children. The relationship between adolescent conception and socioeconomic status is particularly strong at the youngest ages. As suggested above, sexual activity and unwanted conception at 16-18 years of age occur across all social classes, but very early sex and pregnancy occur primarily in situations of serious social and economic deprivation.

Hardy and Zabin (1991) concluded that "the distribution pattern of adolescent births is essentially the same as those for infant mortality, homicide, and violent death among youth, violent crime and illicit drug use, all problems of high prevalence in poor and socially disadvantaged areas" (p. 52). Low educational achievement, persistent poverty, and single-parent status feed into an intergenerational cycle of disadvantage with dismaying "implications for stable family formation and the ability of young parents to provide the nurturing environment and resources necessary for optimal development of their children" (p. 70). Thus, whereas many of the interventions discussed below are needed by all young people in the country as they reach puberty or in the years thereafter, those at highest risk require much more comprehensive, continuing services of an educational, supportive, and medical nature.

COMPARISON WITH OTHER
INDUSTRIALIZED NATIONS

It is only in comparison with similar nations that the magnitude of the adolescent childbearing problem in the United States becomes clear, and it also becomes clear that it could be prevented. In 1986, Jones and colleagues published the results of a study of teenage pregnancy and birth across six Western industrialized nations: the United States, Canada, England and Wales, France, Sweden, and The Netherlands. Of these nations, the United States has by far the highest rates of pregnancy, childbirth, and abortion among its teenagers. In all the other countries, the rates have been steadily declining since 1971; in the United States, the rates declined sharply only until 1976 and since then have shown only a very small decrease. This difference in rates is not attributable only to discrepancies between racial groups; among whites alone, teenage fertility rates are substantially higher in the United States than in any other comparable country. Furthermore, the largest differences exist at the youngest ages. The birth rate to 14-year-olds in the United States, at 5 per 1,000, is four times higher than that in its nearest competitor, Canada. In all countries, the birth rate increases with age through the years to age 20. In other countries, however, a sharp increase in the birth rate is apparent only after the age of 17; among young adolescents, the birth rate increases only slowly. In the United States, by contrast, the birth rate increases steadily from the youngest ages upward, with no distinction in rates of childbearing after the age of 17. Despite easier and more universal access to abortion in other countries, the United States teenage abortion rate is at least as high as the entire teenage pregnancy rate (abortion plus childbearing) in the other five nations, and often higher. Moreover, pregnant or childbearing teenagers in the other countries are more likely to be married.

These differences are not accounted for by different rates of sexual activity, which are much the same across all these nations. It is largely a differential in effective contraceptive practice that accounts for higher pregnancy rates here, a practice that other countries have shown is amenable to intervention (Jones, Forrest, Henshaw, Silverman, & Torres, 1988).

CONCLUSION

American teenagers have higher rates of conception, abortion, and birth than their counterparts in comparable nations. Even high nationwide statistics, however, understate the problem that exists in deprived urban populations, where rates of conception and birth may be twice as high as national averages. Rates of sexual activity changed dramatically in the 1970s and continued to rise in the 1980s, exposing more of the teenage population to the risk of pregnancy. As fewer and fewer teenagers were married, conceptions were more likely to be out of wedlock, and as the practice of "legitimizing" pregnancies declined, more teenage mothers remained single parents. Despite increased use of contraception and the availability of abortion—access to which is becoming more and more difficult for those who cannot afford private care—pregnancy rates to the youngest teenagers have not declined. Although rates of sexual activity have stabilized somewhat, particularly in the black population, young adolescents have changed their sexual behavior the least. Age discriminates between subgroups in the level of their sexual exposure: Gender, racial, and economic differentials in ages of sexual onset are largest in early adolescence and tend to attenuate over the teen years. Similarly, age affects the probability of contraceptive protection once sexual activity is initiated. Therefore the youngest sexually active adolescents are at highest risk of accidental pregnancy, a circumstance leading—despite a high abortion ratio—to unintended birth. Unfortunately those at highest risk in their early teen years live in the poorest areas of our cities, where they are subject to the combined stresses of social, economic, educational, and environmental deprivation.

3

AGE OF SEXUAL ONSET

INTRODUCTION

A young person's age at first coitus has far-reaching implications. Age affects the *context* of sexual activity, its *frequency*, its *nature*, and the quality of the *relationships* within which it occurs. When age is measured not in chronological terms but in terms of years pre- and postpuberty, it affects *fecundity* (or the fertility of partners), hence the risk of pregnancy. Some girls conceive immediately postpuberty, although the risk of conception appears to be higher at a "gynecological" age of 1 or 2 years (Zabin, 1979). A low chronological age at first intercourse increases the risk of adverse effects by extending the *period of sexual exposure*, which not only increases the probability of negative sequelae as a function of time but also increases the *number of partners* to whom a young man or woman is exposed. A low developmental age at first coitus decreases the *probability of effective contraceptive use*, either at that event or over the subsequent years. A pregnancy causes a more profound *disruption of the life cycle* of the mother (or sometimes both parents) the younger she is. Finally, *the impact of interventions* designed to prevent the adverse sequelae of sexual contact will often depend on the ability of young people to respond to them; early adolescents require approaches tailored to their cognitive, educational, and psychological levels. For all these reasons and many more, it is important to understand the correlates of early sexual exposure.

Why do some teenagers engage in sexual activity at or near puberty, while others delay their sexual experiences until later in the teen years? The explanations are many, some of which we will address here. No doubt they include some combination of normative, or social, influences on the one hand, and developmental, distinctly individual, pressures on the other. Young people are subject to personal pressures

27

arising from the process of physical maturation and from their emerging mental and emotional needs. But simultaneously, each individual also experiences the diverse expectations that arise from a specific social context, a context that conveys implicit norms some of which are encouraging, some discouraging, of early sexual contact. How adolescents respond to and integrate the many pressures that come to bear on them has been the subject of considerable research. Debates surround the relationship between puberty and sexual onset, between societal norms and individual behavior, as well as the role of personality and self-concept in mediating these relationships. To what extent hormones, as opposed to socialization, dominate sexual behavior is a central issue; in this chapter, we will discuss insights that recently have begun to illuminate those relationships.

Physical development has more than one kind of influence on sexual onset. Puberty involves hormonal change and thus alters androgen levels—the physiological foundation of the adolescent's sexual timetable. Simultaneously those levels bring about profound changes in the physical and emotional persona of the young person (Billy, Rodgers, & Udry, 1984; Billy & Udry, 1985a, 1985b; Katchadourian, 1980; Smith, Udry, & Morris, 1985; Udry, Billy, Morris, Groff, & Raj, 1985; Udry, Talbert, & Morris, 1986.) Those changes in turn have an effect on the young person's social milieu; physical maturation changes the way teenagers perceive themselves and the way others perceive them. These perceptions influence the expectations, the aspirations, and the opportunities an adolescent experiences during the formative years.

In the meantime, social pressures are also at work. Cultural environment exerts normative pressures on the developing "sexual script" of each individual, a process described by Simon and Gagnon (1986, 1987). They include in this process the development of personal standards of permissiveness and expectations of real and potential sexual relationships. Although they see the internal task of working out that script as inevitably personal and individual, they also see it as an essentially social process; it cannot occur in isolation because it is embedded in a normative context (Simon & Gagnon, 1986). The way an individual adapts to cultural norms creates a classic intersection of biology and society. The relative strength of biological and social influences depends at least in part on the age of the adolescent, chronologically and maturationally, when that process occurs.

We will discuss sexual onset in terms of these competing influences. This discussion would appear to assume that the decision to engage in coitus is the adolescent's own. To the degree that sexual behavior constitutes a series of conscious choices, we can consider sexual onset under the young person's control. In many cases, however, we know that that event was not within a young person's control at all. Moore and colleagues (Moore, Nord, & Peterson, 1989) reported that, especially at young ages, nonvoluntary sexual activity plays a significant role in sexual initiation. This is true throughout the teen years but especially at age 16 and under. Sometimes this initiation involves outright violence, but many other factors or combinations of factors can keep the event from being truly voluntary. Personality, social ambience, and accidental circumstance can come together to make this important event "just happen." But controlled or not, accidental or not, the initiation of coital activity results in a real risk of pregnancy. It often signifies the beginning of sexual behaviors that might otherwise have been postponed. Sexuality, explicit and active, constitutes a new forum in which difficult issues of self-concept and self-esteem must be addressed. Although we need a much better understanding of that initial event, it remains for most young people a marker of developmental importance.

PHYSICAL MATURATION
AND SEXUAL ONSET

In Western, industrialized nations, the age of physical maturity, at least among females, declined over the past century. One clear marker of physical development is menarche, which has a fairly well-documented history in the 19th and 20th centuries (Marshall & Tanner, 1974; Zacharias, Wurtman, & Schatzoff, 1970). The decline in mean age of menarche, constituting as it does a fundamental change in species development, has been rapid: lower by 3 to 4 months every decade until a few generations ago, when it leveled off. For example, an estimate based largely on a white, middle-class sample with a mean age of menarche of 12.6 years indicated that, on average, young women reached menarche 4 months earlier than their mothers (Zacharias et al., 1970).

Research exploring influences on age at menarche has suggested the influence of numerous and diverse factors. Climate, race, culture, nutrition, physical stress, socioeconomic status, and altitude have all been considered. Light, psychosexual stimulation, protein-calorie malnutrition, and other environmental factors have been proposed (Bojlen & Bentzon, 1968; Johnston, 1974; Litt & Cohen, 1973; Roberts & Dann,

1967; Rona & Pereira, 1974). Correlations with skeletal changes (Marshall & Tanner, 1974), secondary sex characteristics (Nicolson & Hanley, 1953), and various measures of body mass, fat, or size (Frisch, 1972; Frisch & Revell, 1971; Johnston, Roche, Schell, & Wettenhall, 1975) have been documented.

Nutritional status, probably protein nutrition, and age of menarche are negatively related on a population basis if not on an individual basis; the better nourished the population, the sooner, on average, young girls reach menarche. This relationship is thought to explain the negative association between socioeconomic status and menarche: The higher the social class, the lower the age at physical maturity. Body mass is also negatively related to age at menarche (Short, 1976), a logical extension of the nutritional relationship. It is possible, however, that this is only an important factor when levels of malnourishment are severely low (Marshall & Tanner, 1974); although some evidence suggests that small differences in body mass may be related to amenorrhea, the relationship between the two is not well established.

It may be, therefore, that nutrition and socioeconomic status mediate the association of race and age at menarche. In fact, racial differences in maturation in the United States disappear when controlled for socioeconomic variables. The negative correlation of social and economic standing with the onset of menses is consistent across nations, despite differences in mean age of menarche (Marshall & Tanner, 1974; Tanner, 1962). Although menarche has occurred earlier, the relative developmental pace of black and white populations in the United States may have changed. Earlier in the century, it was thought that black women reached menarche earlier than white women; now this relationship appears to be reversed. But such differences are small, compared for example with differences between women in the United States and in several of the developing countries of Africa.

Although our interest is not in the specific factors that determine age of menarche, these relationships make it clear that chronological age is not necessarily a good indicator of physical maturation; pubertal age is the relevant measure. The role of hormonal change in sexual behavior, as we shall see, varies as a function of its social context. To one extent or another, however, the interplay between an individual and that context is clearly influenced by physical changes, which have both an internal and external effect and which occur independently of cognitive and emotional maturation. As Short (1976) concluded, although psychological development is related to calendar age, psychosexual development is related to the onset of puberty, controlled by nutritional events.

Pubertal Change

Pubertal development is caused by increasing levels of steroidal hormones. In males, all physical and morphological changes, as well as nocturnal emission and other aspects of maturation, are caused by androgens. In females, estrogens are responsible for morphological changes such as breast development and genital maturation, whereas androgens cause hair growth (Billy & Udry, 1983; Udry et al., 1986). In both sexes, androgens are responsible for increased sex drive experienced during the adolescent years (Pierke, Kockett, & Dittmar 1974; Billy & Udry, 1983). The role of estrogens in sexual motivation is as yet uncertain.

Menarche is a useful marker of female maturation not only because it has a good level of recall reliability but also essentially because there is a strong association between that event and other aspects of sexual development. The ordering of physical manifestations of puberty is fairly constant, with menarche always following peak height velocity, independent of chronological age. In girls, steroid levels start rising between ages 7 and 9 and rise rapidly from the age of 9 until first menstruation (Udry et al., 1986). Because it follows the onset of breast development and the appearance of pubic and axillary hair, and because it is the culmination of years of hormonal change, menarche can be considered to be a late pubertal event. However, because steroidal levels continue to rise throughout the teen years, only reaching adult levels at 18-20 years of age, first menstruation actually occurs early in the process of full physical maturation. Despite the early morphological changes that occur before menarche, breast changes can take 4 to 5 years to complete (Tanner, 1962), and most maturation of the female body takes place after menarche (Udry et al., 1986), affected as it is by continuous exposure to estrogens. Thus, as a measure of the level of sexual maturation, menarche can be seen as occurring fairly late or fairly early in puberty.

A boy's first nocturnal emission may not be as easily recallable an event but has been used with some success as a benchmark in pubertal development. Katchadourian (1980) described it as a late pubertal event; many bodily changes precede it. It is not as clear a marker as is menarche for girls, because all young men may not experience it and, if they do, it may not be their first experience of ejaculation. Its place in the sequence of physical maturation is reasonably well documented, however, and of all the changes a pubertal male experiences, a first "wet dream" is probably the only event that can be dated.

Prepubertal androgen levels are similar in males and females. At puberty, androgens increase by a factor of 5 in females and by a factor of 50 in males. Different androgens are involved in male and female development, primarily testosterone in males and adrenal androgens in females (Apter & Vihko, 1977). After puberty, testosterone levels in males are 8 times higher than those in females, and a free testosterone index (a measure of circulating androgenicity used by Udry and colleagues in studies correlating hormonal levels with sexual behavior) is 100 times higher in males than in females. The adrenal androgens, which are primarily important in female libido, are several times weaker in androgenicity than testosterone.

The decline in mean age of menarche in the modern era means at the very least that all these changes occur at younger ages and that fertility is achieved earlier than before. And when they occur at younger ages, they create a discontinuity between biological maturity, on the one hand, and psychosocial and cognitive development, on the other. We have noted that each of these developmental processes proceeds independently. One effect of earlier physical maturation is to put the young person at greater risk of conception and sexually transmitted diseases before the skills to manage a sexual life are well developed.

One might speculate on the implications of these changes at a population level for the sexual mores of a society. Although the changes in physical maturation in Western society have not been concurrent with the changes in sexual behavior, the effect of declines over a period of 100 years may well have been delayed or prolonged; the possible impact of changes in sexual maturation on current behavior cannot be overlooked if we can document a relationship between puberty and sexual onset.

Puberty and Sexual Onset

Physical development may have become more important in relation to adolescent sexuality as the age of sexual onset declined and probably has its greatest influence among those whose onset is early. Billy and Udry (1983) noted little variation in development by age 16 or 17; most adolescents have reached the final stages. But, as sexual behavior has become earlier, pubertal development has become more important:

Some 13-year-olds have completed most stages of maturation while others have hardly begun.

In several female populations, a positive association has been documented between age of menarche and age of first intercourse (Buck & Stavraky, 1967; Cutler, Garcia, & Krieger, 1979; Udry, 1979; Zabin, Smith, et al., 1986). Zabin, Smith, et al. (1986) documented that relationship among males, as well. There is also a demonstrated association between menarche and first birth, which is evident across cultures (Udry & Cliquet, 1982). The relationship between these two events is inevitably confused by differential contraceptive use, as shown by Presser (1978). Presser also showed that age at menarche is related to age at first birth; because the relationship disappears when controlled for age at first intercourse, she concluded that menarche is not a good predictor of the timing of motherhood. She also showed, however, that age at menarche is related to age at first dating and age at first intercourse. Udry concluded (1979) that "the fact that the relationship between age at menarche and age at first birth disappears when controlled for age at first intercourse is not a proper basis for dismissal of the menarche-birth relationship. Rather, it is evidence that it is through the timing of first intercourse that the relationship comes about" (p. 439).

Udry and colleagues documented the independent effects of androgens on sexual onset by using a free testosterone index and pubertal development to measure hormonal influence and by using age as a residual variable representing social norms, experience, and skills generally learned by chronological age (Billy & Udry, 1985a, 1985b; Smith, Udry, & Morris, 1985). In males, free testosterone levels directly affect coitus, masturbation, and noncoital sexual experience. In females, levels of testosterone are low, and other androgens have direct effects especially on noncoital behavior (Udry, 1979; Udry et al., 1985; 1986). Testosterone appears to work directly on sexual behavior—neither through the perceptions of others dictated by pubertal development nor through age-related norms.

Overall these investigators concluded that the best predictor of sexual behavior is hormonal level rather than age or physical development. For females, however, the effects of hormones are strong for noncoital behaviors but not for intercourse; for males, hormonal effects are strong for both coital and noncoital behavior (Udry et al., 1985). They reported that the differential involvement of females in coitus is more strongly regulated by social processes than by hormones, whereas the differential involvement of males in coitus is primarily controlled by hormones.

The importance of social environment in female behavior has been interpreted to indicate that young women are subject to more controlling social pressures, that they experience more varied normative environments that account for greater differentiation between groups, and/or that they are somehow easier to control (Udry et al., 1986). On the other hand, males are thought to be subject to less control, to experience a more homogeneous and positive normative environment for sexual behavior, and to feel a "more powerful jolt" to their libido from androgens in adolescence. Nonetheless it is reasonable that, even in the presence of different normative environments for sexual behavior, one explanation for gender differences is the impact of androgens on sexual motivation.

Much of the evidence we have about the impact of puberty has been limited to white populations, and less is known about similar associations among black adolescents. Therefore research in an urban school population of black adolescents is enlightening. It was found that the relationship between puberty and first intercourse is particularly strong in the early teens and tends to attenuate over time (Zabin, Smith, et al., 1986). If curves showing ages of menarche for girls and ages of first nocturnal emission for boys are plotted and superimposed on the curves indicating their ages at first intercourse, it is apparent that the two curves have similar shapes; the age of first intercourse for girls lags about 2 years behind the age of menarche, while the age of first intercourse for boys parallels the age of first nocturnal emission (Figure 3.1). The distribution of female puberty is sharply peaked: 75% of the sample reached menarche between the ages of 11 and 13.9 years. This peak is echoed 2 years later by the similar distribution of age at first intercourse. The mean age of menarche is 12.7 years, and that of intercourse is 14.4 years. The distribution of male puberty is wider and peaks at the same age as first intercourse, 13.5 years. The mean age of intercourse, however, is even younger.

The impact of puberty on sexual onset is most evident at the youngest ages, where the differences in rates of sexual activity between maturational groups are the greatest (Figure 3.2). For example, at age 13, nearly 40% of those girls whose menarche occurred at or under 11 years are sexually active; among the middle maturational groups, with menarche at 13 or 14 years of age, about 20%, and 10% among those whose menarche has not yet occurred (menarche at or above 14 years) are sexually active. The differential between early and late maturers does not disappear entirely until age 17. Among the boys at age 11, more than half of those who had their first wet dream at age 11 or under are

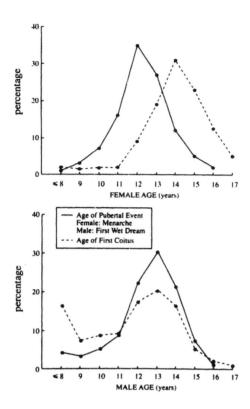

Figure 3.1. Distribution Percentage of Ages of Puberty and Ages of First Coitus Among Black Male and Female Students, 1981 (Reproduced by permission from Zabin et al. *Demography* 23:595-605, 1986. Copyright © Population Association of America.)

sexually active, compared with 40% of those who had it at age 12, and 30% of those who had it at age 13 or 14. Thus, among 12-year-olds, there is a 36 percentage point difference between the earliest and latest maturing males, by age 13 the middle maturational groups have caught up with the earliest group (approximately four out of five are sexually active), and by age 15 the differential has disappeared.

In this group, self-reports reflect relatively early ages of sexual initiation and a substantial amount of prepubertal sex. Among females, 12.7% of first coital events were said to occur before menarche. Among males, 60.7% gave an age of first intercourse that preceded their first

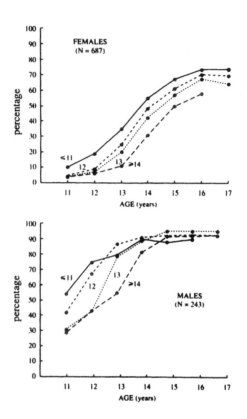

Figure 3.2. Cumulative Percentage of Males/Females Initiating Coitus at Each Age, by Age at First Wet Dream/Menarche

wet dream (Zabin, Smith, et al., 1986); even if we subtract 1 year from the reported age of nocturnal emission to account for its occurrence late in pubertal development (Katchadourian, 1980), it still will appear that 41.4% of the young men describe their first intercourse as prepubertal.

The relationship between age of physical maturation and age of sexual onset tends to disappear when the teenage years are examined as a whole, which masks an association that has important effects on the youngest teenagers. At ages 13 and 14, the relationship is strong; 72% more of the young women with early menarche than of those with late menarche are sexually active. Differentials among males appear at younger ages but disappear earlier. It is therefore in the earliest teen years, years that we shall see are associated with a high risk of unprotected coitus, that pubertal development exerts its greatest influence on sexual onset.

Risk of Pregnancy

On average, even those young women with relatively early sexual onset are 2 to 3 years postmenarche at the time of first coitus (Furstenberg, 1976; Zabin, Kantner & Zelnik, 1979). This allows cycles to have become regular and the adolescent to have become fecund. Although peak fertility is not reached for some young women until a gynecological age of 2 years, conceptions immediately after menarche are unfortunately not rare (Zabin et al., 1979). In fact, the risk of pregnancy is very high at coital onset. A life table analysis of sexually active women aged 18-19 in 1976 showed that one fifth of them become pregnant within 6 months of first sexual intercourse (Zabin et al., 1979). Half of all first premarital teenage pregnancies occur in the first 6 months of sexual activity, and more than one fifth in the first month alone. The risk of another premarital pregnancy is also high among those whose first pregnancy occurs within 6 months of sexual onset. As we shall see, a key factor in explaining the high risk of pregnancy in the first months of sexual activity is age. In the next chapter, we will address some of the reasons behind these relationships; here it is important to note that adolescent subfecundity, which had been thought of as reducing the risk of conception at early ages, is a variable and brief phenomenon and can hardly be relied on as a useful contraceptive.

Prepubertal Sexual Activity

Prepubertal sex is probably a fairly common occurrence in some populations if teenagers' self-reports are credited. The nature and circumstance of these experiences is not well documented, and they therefore represent something of a gap in our understanding of adolescent sexuality. If three out of five inner-city boys in the study cited above reported that they experienced intercourse before nocturnal emission (between ages 6 and 12), and if one in eight inner-city girls reported that she experienced intercourse before menses, the importance of prepubertal sex play as a precursor of pregnancy risk cannot be ignored (Zabin, Smith, et al., 1986). Similar evidence comes from the same students' responses to a set of questions about their first coital event. They were asked the typical question about the age at which they first experienced coitus (had sex, had intercourse, went all the way) and gave the responses that are plotted above. In a later wave of the same study, that question was followed by the query: "When did you first do this after you could really come?" (or for girls, "after your partner could really come?"). Fifty percent of boys and 12% of girls gave a different and later age. Clearly the language with which we explore these subjects, even with the best of care, leaves room for some semantic confusion. But it also would appear that there are precursors of sexual onset that, in many cases, make "first intercourse"—hence first exposure to pregnancy—an event timed not by a change in behavior but rather by a change in developmental status.

Katchadourian (1980) claimed that the primary difference between pre- and postpubescent sexuality is not the capacity to be aroused or to experience orgasm but rather the capacity in males for ejaculation; indeed the physiological capacity for sexual arousal and even for orgasm may be present in both sexes as early as infancy. He said that it is unclear whether physiological responses are similar to those among adults, but "it is during puberty that adult sexual functions emerge. . . . Owing to the immaturity of the prostate gland which produces most of the seminal fluid, prepubescent orgasm in boys (as with females of all ages) does not entail ejaculation" (p. 17). The fact that sexual onset can precede pubertal changes is evidence of the profound impact of environmental and social norms on behavior, regardless of hormonal state. In some settings, physical maturation is obviously not the only or most salient motivator of sexual behavior.

Although our understanding of the interplay of biology and society is not complete, Katchadourian's comment of 1980 is certainly borne out by subsequent research: "It would be something of a marvel if it turned out that endocrine factors had no bearing on the nature and intensity of the sexual drive. Yet almost as certainly we are not about to discover that the intricate machinery of the human mind is driven by some simple 'sex fuel.' . . . (T)he profound hormonal changes in puberty somehow influence the sexual motivation of the adolescent . . . in a psychosocial context, which also determines in crucial ways how the adolescent behaves sexually" (p. 19). Despite many indications that age of puberty and age of first coitus are related, the relationship is often mediated by cultural norms and pressures; thus individual maturational timetables interface with normative behavior patterns in ways that are difficult to separate.

A central question remains whether social or physical influences are more responsible for sexual activity in adolescence. In this context, chronological age can become a marker of social expectation, whereby ambient age norms for sexual activity come to bear increasingly through the teen years as an individual approaches, reaches, and surpasses the age at which sexual activity is expected and/or accepted. The libidinal effects of pubertal change enhance sexual motivation but also change the social pressures and perhaps the opportunities that are available to an individual, as these depend in part on other people's interpretations of the adolescent's "readiness" for sexual behavior. We conclude that "age of puberty exerts an influence separate from that of normative patterns and, when it is low, applies downward pressure on age of sexual onset. . . . (S)ince the risk of early conception is highest among those who start coitus early, the relationship with physical development cannot be ignored" (Zabin, Smith, et al., 1986, p. 604).

CULTURAL NORMS

Despite secular trends that reflect changes on the population level, the maturational factors we have been considering are essentially individual in nature. Cultural norms, on the other hand, represent the influence of the social environment. As suggested above, within the interplay of social and biological forces, hormonal effects are apparently the more potent influences on young men's behavior, and social processes are more important among young women (Billy & Udry, 1985a; Smith, Udry, & Morris, 1985; Udry et al., 1985; Udry et al., 1986). The fact that the social controls that constrain a young woman's sexual behavior reduce hormonal effects on her coital activity is strong evidence of that interplay. Similarly, at older ages, age-related social expectations become proportionately more influential and biological influences less strong. Data on the relationship between puberty and sexual onset indicate that "as age of puberty increases, the cultural influence of social norms, as opposed to the individual developmental timetable, becomes stronger" (Zabin, Smith, et al., 1986, p. 604). The time lag between puberty and sexual onset is not constant, as it would be if biology were equally influential at all ages. It declines with increasing age, under normative pressures, as the probability of coitus within 1 to 2 years of menarche increases dramatically over time.

The impact of social forces on age of sexual onset is also evidenced by broad societal indicators, which show trends that cannot be accounted for by biological factors. We have described the changing norms for sexual behavior in our society: The Kantner and Zelnik surveys of the 1970s gave evidence of how profoundly and rapidly sexual behavior of teenage women changed during those years (Zelnik & Kantner, 1980). The downward pressure on age at first intercourse that occurred during the 1970s was a continuation of a movement toward greater permissiveness that had been going on for decades before. Attitudes changed not only about teenage sexuality but also about premarital and extramarital sex, as well as childbearing out of wedlock. This movement had an impact in all social and economic groups and at all ages, although the largest continuing decrease in age at first intercourse is among white females. Socioeconomic differences, as defined by educational status, are also related to the timing of sexual initiation (Zelnik, Kantner, & Ford, 1981). Differences between subgroups in the sequencing of sexual behaviors, numbers of partners, and frequency of intercourse attest to the impact of social norms on sexual behavior. Young white girls, for example, once initiating coitus, report much higher frequencies of coitus and many more partners than are typically reported by nonwhite teens. Thus, within the broad sweep of behavioral and attitudinal change, social factors discriminate a number of differences between subgroups of the society that cannot be accounted for by differences in physical maturation.

Sexual Scripts

Simon and Gagnon (1986, 1987) have proposed the concept of *sexual scripts* as a way of understanding the process of emerging sexual behavior. The development of an individual's sexual script comes from the interaction of three "scenarios": cultural, interpersonal, and intrapsychic. At the cultural level, social norms exist as guidelines to personal behavior; at the interpersonal level, individuals work out their own sexual scenarios in relation to others; and at the intrapsychic level, each person develops the internal self-motivation on which to act as a sexual being.

To the extent that the cultural scenario weakens and, as in modern society, there is no clear consensus on the appropriate timing and sequencing of sexual behaviors, the need for internal rehearsal becomes stronger. Sexual onset, like other social behaviors, depends on individual adaptation, but its occurrence is more socially influenced than the presence of biological drives would imply. Developing a sexual identity and defining one's own behavioral guidelines remain "in most critical aspects a derivative of the social process" (Simon & Gagnon, 1986, p. 111). Young men and women adopt sexual behaviors at a time that is influenced by hormonal development, but they follow a script that is largely determined by social expectations.

Transitional Behaviors

In an important longitudinal study, Jessor and Jessor (1977) examined the initiation of sexual intercourse as one transitional behavior among many. They embedded the sexual behavior of teenagers in the overall experience of these years, holding that many of the "problem" behaviors of adolescence are simply behaviors that are subject to age-graded norms and therefore, "when engaged in earlier, depart from the regulatory age norms defining what is appropriate at that age or stage in life" (p. 42). Sexual activity is preeminently one of those behaviors.

Personality, perceived social context, and behavior develop with regularities across the transitions. The initiation of drinking, smoking marijuana, and sexual onset are correlated with changes in attitude and personality. The timing of these changes differs for those whose transitional behaviors occur at different ages, but regularities in development remain and show the greatest magnitude of change in early adolescence. Changes in attitude that are often associated with transitional behaviors include a decline in the value placed on achievement and a decline in religiosity, increased value on independence, social criticism, and more tolerance of deviance. Simultaneous changes in the young person's perceived environment may include declining parental control and increasing friends' approval for—and engagement in—problem behaviors. Although conventional behaviors decline, the resultant behaviors can include increased drinking, sexual experience, drug use, and general deviance.

Although not universal, these are salient aspects of developmental change in the transition phase of adolescence. Jessor and Jessor (1977) concluded that many changes they explored "are in the direction that is socially defined as more mature" (p. 162). Because problem behavior is often age graded within our culture and because behaviors that are forbidden to minors may even be allowable at older ages, they may actually define adulthood. Thus "problem proneness has many attributes that may well be seen as 'maturity proneness,' and the changes we have been describing may perhaps be taken as part of coming of age in America" (p. 162).

Jessor and Jessor interpreted their data to support the interpretation of these activities as markers of a transition in psychosocial status, not merely as the adoption of new behaviors. Sexual onset may be seen as evidence of a coherent developmental change within individual adolescents. The study does not address a correspondence between those changes and cognitive and emotional maturity, but it identifies a pattern of developmental change that is coordinated with the timing of certain behaviors. Groups that make various transitions at different times tend to converge developmentally by the end of the transitional years. This suggests a "catch up" phenomenon in psychosocial development, as occurs in physical development.

The idea that early sexual onset is part of a global transition to adult behaviors is not incompatible with the idea that at young ages it is accompanied by immature cognitive constructs and emotional capacities. The conclusion that "problem proneness can often mean no more than developmental precocity" (Jessor & Jessor, 1977, p. 248), which may revolve around early physical maturation, may suggest that differences in timing "wash out" in the long run. Because these years represent a developmentally complex period, however, the price that is paid when events occur out of synchrony may be considerable. Therefore, as we shall see in the following chapter, discontinuities in development have serious implications for the management of sexuality in the adolescent years.

Clustering of Behaviors

Another approach to sexual onset suggests that premature sexual behavior is one of a number of risk behaviors to which certain "types" of individuals are prone. However, there are many possible reasons why behaviors of certain kinds often appear together, reasons that may be social, psychological, developmental, or ecological. The work of Jessor and Jessor indicates that problem behaviors in the teenage years tend to cluster; more than one socially unacceptable or self-destructive behavior is likely to be exhibited by the same individual. Some of these behaviors, such as early sexual activity, are only problematic because they occur at young ages; others are problematic whenever they occur.

And many young people who engage in early sexual contact exhibit no other "risk" behaviors and manage their sexual contacts responsibly. The notion that other characteristics identify an early sexual onset "type" was recurrent in the academic literature for some time. In 1973, Sorenson described the "adventurer" who was more casual in relationships, less concerned with love and more with ego satisfaction, more in conflict with parents, more permissive, and lower in responsibility and self-esteem. Those who fit this description had more partners and a higher frequency of intercourse in the month prior to interview; 75% of them were age 15 or younger at first intercourse, compared with 51% of the monogamous sample. Only 20% of the girls in the study group fell in this category, and differences in age were small; many early starters could not be identified in this way. Schofield (1965), in England in the 1960s, found that early starters left school in greater numbers and came more often from working-class homes and less often from religious homes. He described a different pattern of sexual activity in this group, with first intercourse being less often at home, more often for "no reason," and less often for "love."

These studies are largely descriptive, not explanatory. Even if behaviors or characteristics tend to cluster, the explanations for these associations can be many. Developmental, environmental, and social factors may all interact to produce a high-risk behavioral profile in some teenagers. Ample evidence supports the existence of these patterns. The relationship between problem behaviors of different kinds can be important in identifying at-risk populations and in designing interventions for them. In a study of clinic patients, Zabin (1984) found a strong negative correlation between smoking levels and sexual onset. Particularly among white women, those who initiate coitus at a very early age report smoking levels that exceed the national average for adults, even though the mean age of the study cohort was barely 16 years. This relationship holds for young black women too, although levels of smoking are substantially higher among whites. Relationships between a substance "index" and sexual onset were explored among urban youth (Zabin, Hardy, Smith, & Hirsch, 1986). They do not hold when considered across gender/race groups; for example, young black males have the earliest sexual onset but the lowest levels of substance use. But *within* each gender/race group, the younger the adolescent at first coitus, the higher his or her substance use index.

Peer Influence

Peers exert powerful social pressures on teenagers. Smith and colleagues (Smith, Udry, & Morris, 1985) looked at the relative influence of pubertal development and friends' behavior on the sexual involvement of teenagers. They found that, for males and females, both the young person's level of physical maturation and the sexual involvement of his or her best friend are related to sexual motivation. Once again, social effects are stronger for young women than for young men. At lower levels of libidinal motivation, young women are less influenced by their friends' behavior; at higher levels of maturation, friends' behavior becomes a more important influence. Among young men, greater maturation and more sexual activity among friends both have a positive effect on sexual involvement, with the effect of friends being somewhat stronger.

Because a young person's stage of pubertal development affects the way he or she is perceived by others, it also affects the young person's perception of self. That self-perception in turn influences the adolescent's selection of peers, who then have an independent effect on social behavior (Smith, 1989). Because both physical characteristics and self-image affect the way others relate to him or her, they may affect the opportunities that are open to the adolescent to engage in high-risk behaviors. Thus the biological time clock helps create the adolescent's social world but is not equally dominant in all settings. Its effects are weakest when social restraints are strongest; when the social setting is permissive, libidinal development and friends' behavior have more direct and obvious effects (Smith, 1989).

It is a normal part of the developmental process for the teenager to relate increasingly to peers and less to parents than at younger ages. In that context, the values of the adolescent will come to accord more with those of his or her peers and often to become more permissive in that process. It would appear that that process is somewhat accelerated for those whose sexual onset is early, which may short-circuit one of the tasks of adolescence—the development of a personal standard of behavior. In that case, the presence of a sexually active peer group can have a greater impact on youthful behavior than it might have a few years later.

Family Influence

In American society, the family is considered to be the appropriate institution to give moral guidance and to promote healthy behavior among its children. Unfortunately, even if parents are well equipped to provide moral support and values to their children, they are not always the best or most willing providers of guidance in the area of sexual behavior. Some lack the information to do so. Others are afraid to deal with matters with which they themselves are uncomfortable. All too often, social and economic pressures lessen the family's ability to protect the younger child or to equip the older child for the larger environment. And in some extreme circumstances, it may even be that within the family setting itself a young girl is most at risk of unintended or unwanted intercourse.

Even without the problems of limited knowledge, economic pressures, and problem relationships, parents and teenagers often find it awkward to discuss sexual subjects. Communication with peers or even sexual partners is difficult at best, particularly for young adolescents; with parents, it may be prohibitive. The desire to keep this part of life private is easy to understand, especially when sexual activity is an expression of the natural process of separation from parental control. Nor is this reticence peculiar to American youth; it is observed in more open and less ambivalent societies such as Sweden (Jones et al., 1986).

It is difficult to assess the impact of family communication on adolescent sexuality when the various ways in which family influence are expressed are not well understood. Researchers have not always found the strong correlation between parent-child communication and sexual onset that societal attitudes would lead one to expect; there is generally less effect than they hypothesize. Studies are impeded by the difficulty of assessing the *quality* of communication. Even data on the *quantity* of discussion are open to question, because parents and children have very different perceptions of the level of communication that has taken place between them. When asked whether discussion of a specific topic has ever taken place between parent and child, the parent will often maintain that it has; the son or daughter, that it has not (Smith, Zabin, & Hirsch, 1985). This phenomenon may be of more than methodological importance; it may suggest the level of explicit discourse that is necessary if parents' oral communications are to have a real impact on their offspring's attitudes and behavior.

Despite these difficulties, can we say anything about parental communication as a determinant of adolescent sexual behavior? Solid studies of this aspect of adolescents' lives are rare. There is some evidence that adolescents who perceive communication with their parents to be poor are more likely to initiate a range of risk behaviors early (Jessor

& Jessor, 1977). However, the relationship between parental communication and adolescent behavior is elusive. For example, girls whose mothers report discussing sex with them are less likely to initiate coitus, but when the daughters' own reports are considered, this relationship disappears (Newcomer & Udry, 1985). Here, too, mothers and daughters are not in agreement on the level of communication that has taken place. Early starters are no more likely to communicate with their parents despite long exposure to pregnancy, and if they do, it is difficult to determine whether discussion preceded or followed sexual onset.

In a small retrospective study of young black women, Evans (1987) found that perceived attitudes of female friends, fathers, mothers, and teachers discriminated between childbearing, sexually active, and virgin groups, with the young mothers perceiving the least disapproval of sexual involvement and childbearing. Because the subjects were questioned after their own sexual initiation or childbirth, it is impossible to determine whether these differences preceded the adolescents' behaviors and choices; only a follow-up of those not sexually active could evaluate changes in the attitudes of significant others, perceived or real, that occur with a teenager's changing circumstance. Nevertheless two interesting points emerged. Fathers' attitudes both toward sexual involvement and childbearing were perceived as strongly negative by all groups but particularly by those who were not sexually active. Childbearers perceived mixed messages from their teachers and mothers, who they thought were supportive of childbearing but not of sexual activity. These perceptions suggest how hard it is to elucidate the role of family attitudes in adolescent sexual behavior.

Other family factors associated with higher risk of early childbearing may also reflect a situation in which parental control and communication are difficult. It may be that behavioral manifestations of child-parent interaction are symptoms of underlying emotional relationships that may be characterized by closeness and identification or by alienation and rejection. Furthermore the desire *not* to communicate is not necessarily indicative of weak parental ties; it may represent just the opposite—a desire to spare parents what their offspring believe will hurt or disturb them. Thus communication *and* the nature of the emotional ties underlying communication are both difficult to define and measure.

It is not entirely surprising that the direct effects of parental communication on the timing of sexual onset are weak. Those adolescents most in need of support and counsel are likely to be those whose thinking accords least with their parents and is most influenced by peers. That is not to imply, however, that indirect effects of the family setting on the young person are not powerful influences at every stage of development. At an individual level, family relations have an important impact on the young person's emerging self-concept, aspirations, and expectations for the future; it is through the family that they learn to understand the effects of their own behavior. Therefore, however limited the impact of direct verbal communication on sexual onset may be, the role of the family as a socializing institution, even a socializing institution in the specific area of sexual behavior, should not be minimized.

Parental effects may not operate primarily through oral communication or may occur entirely separate from verbal exchange. It has been found that a similarity between a mother's and daughter's ages of coital onset is better explained by similarity of age at menarche than by level of communication about sex. This suggests a biological rather than an attitudinal connection between mothers and daughters in their sexual behavior (Newcomer & Udry, 1984).

Social control, such as that exerted through curfews, limits placed on an adolescent's independence, the regulation of free time, and the supervisory presence of parents may exert important effects. For example, Hogan and Kitagawa, in a study of fertility in black adolescents in Chicago (1985), found that lax parental control of dating was one of the factors associated with a high risk of teenage pregnancy. Being in a nonintact family or in one with five or more siblings, situations that inevitably put greater strain on parental resources, were also associated with increased risk of early pregnancy. In some cases, curfews and similar limits can represent elements in a conflictual parent-child relationship, not aspects of control or communication (Boxill, 1987).

The family, important as it is, does not act in isolation. It is only one of a triad of contexts that provide the major influences of childhood and adolescence. The relative influence of each component of the triad varies through infancy, childhood, and into adolescence (Hardy & Zabin, 1991). The school and the community have increasing impact on development as the child grows. In infancy, the family is paramount; an infant depends almost entirely on the immediate environment for safety and affection. Although day care is becoming a common context for the care of infants and young children, the range of a child's contacts in the preschool years is still narrow. Optimal growth and development depend on the household alone. As the child enters school, his or her contacts widen; some of the family's influence is superseded by the social environment of the school. At this stage, the impact of the community at large generally remains minimal. As the child reaches adolescence, however, the range of his or her acquaintance and experience expands; the influence of the family gives way somewhat to that of the community as well as the school, both of which are embodied in the young person's peers. Normally, however, even though the individual increasingly differentiates him- or herself as an independent person, the family remains an important influence throughout adolescence.

This pattern—the gradual intrusion of broader influences into the sphere of a strong and sustained family—is less common a pattern in areas of urban poverty. In these areas, relatively few families are intact, and single mothers must often struggle to provide basic necessities for their children. Subject to the multiple stresses of poverty and deprivation, often tied to low-paying jobs with difficult hours, parents may have little time and energy for children. Inevitably children are often without supervision, and the overall influence of family life is diminished.

As family cohesion and stability break down, the ability of parents to interact with the adolescent diminishes. It becomes difficult to establish limits in a weak family context and to reward socially acceptable behavior while censuring undesirable behavior. Parental control can be lost at the very time when the community is becoming more influential. In this circumstance, the characteristics of the community become a central influence on adolescent development, and if the nature of the community is conducive to maladaptive behavior, the results can be predictable.

The Community

When we look at the geographic distribution of adolescent childbearing in an urban setting, we see it focused in disadvantaged areas, areas in which symptoms of poverty, ill health, and risk behaviors are also prevalent. Why should geographic environment have so great an impact on individual behaviors? Scholars debate the processes by which communities exert their effects, and suggest alternative explanations, all of which may play a role. The culture of poverty may impinge on the young person through the weakened institutional structures that serve him or her (poor schools, poor health delivery systems, etc.), through the social contacts that perpetuate the means through which others have adapted to the same settings, or through social contagion in which the growing child is "exposed" to risk. Although the sociological explanation of this phenomenon is not our subject, these effects are indeed powerful. Unfortunately, families in the most disadvantaged neighborhoods are likely to have the fewest resources with which to protect their children from negative influences. Although clearly influential in determining a young person's perception of possibility, their role is often weakened by the opportunity structure and the expectations of the community in which they live.

In fact, many of the effects of the environment work *through* the family. The cultural milieu plays an important role in determining parental attitudes and beliefs about education, employment, and religion, all of which influence the options and opportunities experienced by a child or adolescent. The kinds of family resources that are available are influenced by the cultural and economic environment, not just by circumstances of the family itself. And the life-style of parents will have a strong influence on the range of choices perceived by children; it may intensify the effect of the community rather than protect the adolescent from them.

Economic prospects, human services, and living conditions all have an impact on adolescent development. Housing quality and population density will often determine to which elements of human life a child or adolescent is exposed, as they limit privacy for parents and children. Opportunities for employment, day care, and transportation can all impact a family's potential standard of living. Human services and resources, such as quality education, recreation, and accessible medical care, also contribute to the quality of the family's life. Prospects for employment and patterns of family formation that surround a child during the formative years inevitably structure and define his or her own motivation, expectations, and achievement.

Unfortunately, in poor urban areas, many of the most adverse conditions in family, in school, and in the community coincide. The influence of peers becomes compelling in the teen years, and the family cannot exert the positive influence needed to protect a young person from dangerous behaviors around him or her. Schools in these areas are understaffed and have few resources relative to the needs of the high-risk populations they serve. Hogan and Kitagawa (1985) described that high-risk situation in the poorest areas of Chicago. They found that teenagers from environments that combine six specific risk factors—lower class, a ghetto neighborhood, nonintact families, five or more siblings, a sister who is a teenage mother, and lax parental control of dating—have pregnancy rates eight times that of girls from settings with none of these risk factors.

Clearly, early sexual onset and the problems associated with it are not restricted to these settings. The national statistics cited in Chapter 2 give evidence that coital activity by the midteen years is widespread. Nor does early onset necessarily imply a breakdown in family relationships. Numerous and pervasive messages suggest to the adolescent that this is expected behavior; to countermand those influences requires strong and positive messages from the family and the community. In whatever directions their influences tend, the role of family and environment in creating situations of risk must inform our assessments of adolescents who engage in, and adolescents who resist, the pressures around them.

THE ROLE OF SELF-CONCEPT

However powerful external influences may be, within the limits set by the family and the larger community there remains an important role for the individual. External determinants of development have a different impact on different individuals; they may even vary in their impact on the same individual at different times in the life cycle. A single cultural and familial setting does not give rise to homogenous sexual behaviors. The wide variation in timing of sexual onset that occurs in similar circumstances points to the importance of the individual in integrating and transforming his or her experience. Ultimately sexual choices are filtered through the individual, however strong ambient pressures may be.

Within a social environment, each adolescent perceives certain costs and benefits of sexual activity. Bauman and Udry (1981) proposed an econometric model of sexual behavior along these lines; each person computes a personal equation of utilities and costs of sexual relations. They attribute very early onset among black males to higher expectations of positive utility, or "higher subjective expected utility," of sexual onset than among white adolescent males. A similar model of decision making in relation to contraceptive use was proposed by Luker (1975), combining expected positive and negative outcomes of a behavior with the subjective expectancy that the outcome will occur. However, defining all the costs and benefits of sexual activity which individuals perceive is difficult, particularly as some are hidden or unconscious. Moreover a young person's estimate of the probability of each consequence is intensely subjective and likely to change over time (Morrison, 1985).

Aspirations and expectations for the future have also been postulated as important determinants of the decision to start coital activity (Furstenberg, 1976; Hayes, 1987; Mott & Marsiglio, 1985). Adolescent images of the future are determined in part by the perceptions a young person has of him- or herself; these perceptions are influenced by the system of rewards that surround each person. Hofferth (1987) proposed that reward structures influence young people's sexual activity by determining how they evaluate the consequences of certain behaviors. Educational motivation, for example, is associated with later coital activity, higher contraceptive use, and higher rates of abortion if pregnancy occurs. The value placed on education is related to cognitive structures and prior achievements; in this way, higher aspirations are logically connected with self-esteem. Recent emphasis on the role of self-esteem in adolescent behavior reflects the hope that individuals can compensate for detrimental social circumstance. The findings connecting self-esteem directly with sexual initiation are mixed. There is no clear evidence that low self-esteem is connected with early sexual onset, contraceptive use, or childbearing (Hayes, 1987); in fact, by some measures, self-esteem is higher among those with early coitus. Although personality variables such as self-esteem and locus of control are correlated with contraceptive use, their effects are small and limited to specific situations (Morrison, 1985). The relationship of self-esteem with the timing of first coitus and pregnancy must depend on the meaning of those events in the cultural context surrounding the adolescent.

Although many studies have analyzed the components of decision making about contraception, there is a notable dearth of similar information when it comes to the decision to engage in intercourse. As long ago as 1975, Bernard wrote, "It is interesting to note that in all the schemata for developmental stages in women, based as they are almost exclusively on childbearing, so little attention has been paid to the importance of sexual initiation, despite the stress society has long put on the maintenance of virginity" (Bernard, 1975, p. 244). Perhaps there is a recognition today that, whereas childbearing affects the society as a whole, "virginity" is a more private concern. It is the association of early sexual initiation with both abortion and childbearing, however, that makes it critical that we explore its correlates.

CONCLUSION

How shall we understand early sexual onset? If our description is not to be completely deterministic, the individual must remain the crucible in which pressures and restraints from a number of sources are integrated.

Thus our attempts to analyze the numerous influences on sexual onset must be informed by an image of the young person as an interactive agent who retains the ability to resist the pressures of society or even of his or her own hormones. This process is summarized in Figure 3.3. The long intergenerational history leading to a specific moment of choice is represented on the left. The social, economic, and cultural influences passed on to the adolescent through family, peers, and the norms of the community will have affected each teenager's sense of self, aspirations and expectations for the future, and ability to utilize prior experience to address current and future decisions. Similarly, developmental events will determine not only the young person's libidinal drives but also his or her ability to resist those biological forces. When the opportunity for sexual initiation arises, the process that the adolescent is engaged in, consciously or not, is part of a historic dynamic. The decision, however, must be made in the context of the immediate developmental moment; the only cognitive, emotional, and experiential resources available to the adolescent are those that he or she has already acquired. And those will necessarily be limited by chronological age and developmental status. The right side of the model represents the influences on the adolescent at the moment when the opportunity for sexual intercourse is present, an opportunity that may itself be a product of the same developmental and normative forces. These include family, peers, and the community around him or her, a community whose perception of the adolescent is affected by his or her own self-image. Because we do not see that individual as powerless, we recognize the possibility that individual intervention may help change a young person's calculus of choice. But because we see the influences on the adolescent as powerful and pervasive, we recognize how extensive that intervention must be.

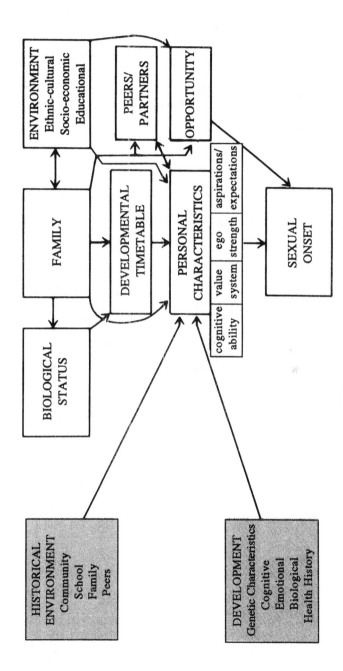

Figure 3.3. Model Depicting Influences on the Onset of Coitus and Interactions Between Them

53

4

ADOLESCENT SEXUAL BEHAVIOR AND CONTRACEPTIVE USE

INTRODUCTION

If the developmental age of an adolescent at the time of sexual initiation has a profound impact on her future life, it is largely because of its effects on the ways in which she understands and manages her sexuality. We have seen that, in early adolescence, discontinuities between physical development and emotional, psychological, and cognitive development are likely to be most pronounced. Her ability to comprehend the consequences of her behaviors, to form stable relationships, to communicate effectively with a partner, or to seek protective counsel may be immature whatever her hormones tell her—or tell the world about her. Thus, even when sexual onset is a matter of "choice," the young person may be as unprepared for it as if it were involuntary or coerced. The younger she is, the more problematic each aspect of sexual life may be and the higher the probability that she will experience detrimental consequences from her sexual behavior. Because many of the normal characteristics of adolescents have a pervasive influence on the way they manage their sexuality, it is not the exceptional teenager but virtually every sexually active teenager (or almost sexually active teenager) who experiences the kinds of problems we address in this chapter.

We will examine the ways in which adolescents form relationships, the place of sexual intercourse within those relationships, and barriers that hinder protective behavior, against the background of normal adolescent cognitive and psychological capacities. We will explore discrepancies between their abstract knowledge and their attitudes and behaviors. Although there is debate about the weight that can be attributed to various influences on adolescent development and about the flexibility or rigidity of the stages through which they pass, there is little disagreement that young people complete certain developmental tasks in a predictable sequence, albeit at different chronological ages. Without accomplishing each task, it is assumed that an adolescent cannot achieve—or will have difficulty achieving—the capacities that are utilized at a subsequent stage. We will not attempt here to add to the large literature on the psychological development of adolescents but rather will focus on well-described developmental constructs that appear relevant to the management of their sexual lives.

THE NATURE OF
ADOLESCENT SEXUAL ACTIVITY

What do we mean when we speak of adolescents' sexual activity as "risk" behavior? We mean that because of the ways in which they frequently manage their relationships, they are at risk of pregnancy and sexually transmitted disease. We mean that there is evidence that their health, their education, and their economic or social well-being may be put in jeopardy. We mean that the nature of their relationships may be exploitative (or permit them to be exploited) and therefore damaging to themselves or to others. And we mean that whatever positive purposes their sexual behavior serves for them—and it does indeed serve some positive purposes, or else they would not pursue it—it represents at some level a psychosocial, emotional, or physical threat to their healthy development into adulthood.

What is the nature of adolescents' sexual behavior? What is it that puts them at risk of negative consequences? Do aspects of their behavior *protect* them against risk? How does the management of their sexual lives relate to the ways normal teens are expected to think, feel, and behave?

- On the whole, teenagers have *low frequencies of intercourse* both in absolute terms and in comparison to adult populations. The modal, or most common, response among teenagers when asked how many times they had intercourse in the last month is zero (Zelnik & Kantner, 1977), even when asked at the time of a contraceptive clinic visit (Zabin & Clark, 1981). Even during the most sexually active month in their experience, teenage women in the clinic study report a modal frequency of only two acts of intercourse. Frequency of intercourse is particularly low in the first months following sexual onset, with a higher expected frequency being typical of first-time clinic visitors (Zabin & Clark, 1981). In general, sexually active white girls have higher frequencies of coitus than black girls, a difference not accounted for by age.

Sexually active males aged 15-19 report a mean of only 2.7 acts of intercourse in the last 4 weeks (Sonenstein et al., 1991), ranging from 1.8 among 15-year-olds to 3.5 among 19-year-olds. In a year, teenagers have intercourse half as often as 18- to 29-year-olds (35 compared with 78 acts of intercourse) (Smith, 1991).

Periods of abstinence are frequent. For example, in a study of first-time visitors to a family-planning clinic, 44% of the sexually active teenage women reported periods of abstinence lasting at least 4 months, with a new period of exposure beginning 3 to 3½ months prior to the clinic visit (Zabin & Clark, 1981). In another study, one in five sexually active 15- to 19-year-old females had not had intercourse in the last 3 months (Forrest & Singh, 1990). Sexually active males in the same age group spend, on average, half the year with no sexual partner. The younger they are, the longer the periods of abstinence: Among 15-year-olds, it is nearly 8 months; among 19-year-olds, 4.3 months (Sonenstein et al., 1991).

- Teenage *sexual relationships are episodic* in nature. Even when adolescents see themselves as "monogamous," relationships may be short-lived and sequential. Therefore they are very likely to have many partners in the course of their teen years, especially when their first coital experiences are at young ages.

Although multiple partners are common among teenagers, they are usually in the context of sequential monogamous relationships, not simultaneous sexual partnerships. Sexually active teenage men report, on average, 2 different sexual partners in the last 12 months (Sonenstein et al., 1991), but only 20% report more than 1 partner within the same month. Nevertheless teenage males report an average of 5 sexual partners since first intercourse, with differences among subgroups (11.3 among blacks, 5.2 among whites) accounted for largely by differences in age of onset. Those with very early onset are most likely to have multiple partners: At the age of 15, sexually experienced young men already report an average of 4.1 sexual partners (6.4 among blacks, 3.5 among whites) (Sonenstein et al., 1991). Data on young women are less specific, but sexually active white females report many more partners than do black females

(Zabin & Clark, 1981). Approximately 58% of sexually active 15- to 19-year-old females have had 2 or more sexual partners, as have 71% of 20- to 24-year-olds (Forrest & Singh, 1990). Sonenstein and colleagues (Sonenstein et al., 1991) concluded: "Among adolescents, having more than one partner in a year is generally not a sign of a 'sexual adventurer' but of the instability of monogamous adolescent relationships. A typical picture of an adolescent male's year would be separate relationships with two partners, lasting a few months each, interspersed with several months without any sexual partner" (p. 166).

- Adolescents are *less likely to use contraception at first intercourse* the younger they are at that event and less likely to seek prompt assistance in the choice of a method. Even when they adopt a contraceptive method, they are less likely than older teenagers and young adults to use it consistently and effectively. As discussed in Chapter 2, despite improved levels of contraceptive use by young men and women at first intercourse (Forrest & Singh, 1990; Sonenstein et al., 1989), a large proportion are still unprotected at that event; the younger they are, the more likely they are to use an ineffective method or no contraception at all. Among teenage women in 1988, 65% used a contraceptive method at first intercourse. Because 56% used a method requiring male involvement (withdrawal or condom), communication with a partner is essential; 35% still used no method (Forrest & Singh, 1990). In data from 1965 to 1988, Mosher and McNally (1991) found that 60% of those whose age of sexual onset was under 15 years used no method of contraception at first intercourse, compared with 44% of those 19 years or older. Much of the difference was due to increased use of the pill in older groups. Those between ages 15 and 18 were most likely to use the condom, while those under age 15 were least likely to use the condom *and* least likely to use the pill.

The difference in contraceptive use according to age of onset is also apparent in Sonenstein's data on adolescent males (1989). In 1988, at first intercourse 79% of those under age 12 at sexual onset used no contraception or an ineffective method; this proportion dropped to 61% of 12- to 14-year-olds, 33% of 15- to 17-year-olds, and 12% of 18- to 19-year-olds. Furthermore, improvements noted in comparison to 1979 are least apparent in the youngest groups.

On average, teenagers who visit a doctor or clinic for contraception do so 11 months after sexual onset (Zelnik, Koenig, & Kim,

1984), but this interval is much longer among young teens. In a study of girls at 32 family planning clinics, those with onset at age 15 and under delay a mean of 23.5 months before attending, compared with 10.6 months among those with onset at ages 16-19 (Zabin & Clark, 1981).

These periods of delay increase the risk of conception inordinately because of the large proportion of risk that occurs in the early months of exposure, a risk that is highly correlated with age at first intercourse (Zabin et al., 1979; Zabin, 1981). Because levels of contraceptive protection vary positively with age, and because the use of contraception tends not only to lower risk but to distribute it more evenly over time, the proportion of risk experienced by the youngest adolescents in early exposure is particularly high. When they delay their clinic attendance, they are very likely to show up at a contraceptive clinic only when they have already conceived.

• Sexually active teens are *unlikely to receive timely treatment for sexually transmitted diseases* and are unlikely to recognize their need for that treatment. They are at higher risk of STDs than any other age group. For example, among sexually active females, rates of gonorrhea are highest in the 10-14 and 15-19 age groups, at 3,500 cases per 100,000 sexually active females (DiClemente, 1990). Sexually active adolescents similarly have the highest rates of syphilis and chlamydia in the population; rates of STDs decline exponentially past age 19 (Bell & Holmes, 1984). Minority groups are at even higher risk; for example, among blacks aged 15-19, the age-adjusted gonorrhea rate is 15 times higher than among whites in the same age group. The epidemiological evidence, DiClemente concluded, suggests that "a substantial proportion of adolescents engage in high risk behavior associated with the acquisition and transmission of STDs" (1990, p. 11).

In addition to length of exposure and multiple partners, biological and psychological attributes of adolescents put them at increased risk. Adolescent women are more susceptible to STDs due to immature histological structure of the vaginal epithelium, which is more prone to infection (Cates & Rauh, 1985). Psychologically, denial and a feeling of immunity contribute to unprotected sexual behavior and cause both exposure to and denial of these diseases.

Of course, concern about STDs is particularly acute due to the AIDS epidemic, in which adolescents are emerging as a high-risk group. Lesions from STDs increase that risk. Unfortunately this new risk is concurrent with federal cutbacks that have made it increasingly difficult for family planning clinics to meet the needs arising from the STD epidemic (Althaus, 1991).

• Adolescent women *may not recognize or acknowledge pregnancy promptly* and thus limit their access to safe abortion or early prenatal care. During the 1980s, a declining proportion of childbearing 15- to 19-year-olds received first trimester care (Hayes, 1987). Risk factors for inadequate prenatal care (no care at all or no care until the third trimester) include coming from a low-income background, being young, nonwhite, unmarried, and having completed fewer than 12 years of schooling (Singh, Torres, & Forrest, 1985); and all of these are often characteristics of the childbearing teen. In a Baltimore study, for example, among teenagers registering for prenatal care, those aged 15 or under registered on average at 18.2 weeks gestation, compared with an average gestation of 16.5 weeks among those aged 16 or over (Hardy & Zabin, 1991).

Nationally, in 1986, 76% of infants in the United States were born to mothers who began prenatal care in the first trimester of pregnancy, over 80% of those whose mothers were ages 25-39. Among 15- to 19-year-olds, however, the proportion with first trimester care was only 53%; among those under age 15, 36%. Similarly 6.6% of mothers under age 15 and 3.8% of those aged 15-19 received no care at all, compared with an average across all ages of 1.9%. White teenagers are less likely to receive adequate prenatal care than black teenagers, although in women over age 20, the reverse is true (Brown, 1989).

Teenagers consistently have abortions later in pregnancy than older women. Nearly half of all abortions after 12 weeks are in teenagers, who are twice as likely as older women to obtain abortions after the first trimester (Cates, 1980). Their tendency to deny, delay, or have difficulty obtaining an abortion is associated with longer gestation; of abortions performed at 13-15 weeks, 70% more occurred among teenagers than older women; over 16 weeks gestational age, 100% more occurred among teenagers (Cates, 1980). The younger the teenager, the more likely she is to have a later abortion: In 1977, 23% of abortions to those age 14 and under were second trimester, compared with 12% at ages 15-19 and 8% at ages 20 and over. Such delays contribute to the risks experienced by teenagers undergoing abortion. When adjusted for gestational age, teenagers have lower morbidity and mortality from induced abortion than older women (Cates et al., 1983). Due to increasing risks with the duration of the pregnancy, however, the tendency to delay has the largest single effect on teenagers' risks of complications. Most of these characteristics of adolescent sexual behavior clearly tend to put them at increased risk. But it is a risk that they are not cognitively or emotionally able to appreciate. Elkind (1967) described the adolescent's construction of what he calls a *personal fable,* characterized by a belief in the invincibility of self, a feeling of being unique and therefore not liable to the risks that pertain to one's peers. Such a belief may result in the adoption of risk behaviors in an apparent disregard for others and often in choices that appear "irresponsible." Elkind placed this egocentric phase of development in early adolescence, which has implications for the ability of those adolescents who initiate coitus early to adopt self-protective behavior. The observation that adolescents often act as if they are "immune" to pregnancy is consistent with Elkind's description: If they see themselves as "different," neither abstract knowledge nor the observed experience of others translates into an accurate perception of personal risk. The following sections will address other developmental characteristics related to their behaviors, with the hope that an understanding of the association of development and risk will suggest the form that optimal intervention might take.

ADOLESCENT PERCEPTIONS OF THEIR PARTNERS AND SEXUAL SELVES

Adolescent Relationships

Adolescents' relationships are characterized by instability; the youngsters juxtapose intense "love" partnerships with casual partnerships and often have difficulty telling them apart. Eriksen (1965), in describing the adolescent phase of identity formation, noted that youngsters at these ages are unable to form stable attachments because they do not have stable self-images. The "crushes" or love relationships of early adolescence are an attempt to achieve identity and are not primarily sexual in motivation.

Constructing and strengthening a consistent idea of self are key developmental themes in adolescence. Eriksen spoke of the development of an "identity" or stable self-concept as the primary task of adolescence and proposed that the early latency period, during which social controls are internalized, lays an essential foundation for ego development. Before a stable sense of self is established, it is difficult to make crucial decisions about the future or to form reliable bonds with others. If the tasks of this early period are incomplete, then role diffusion and lack of commitment, which frequently mark adolescence, can be intensified.

Ego development in its various stages also has an impact on interpersonal style and the potential for establishing relationships. In an early, preconformist phase, individuals may be "wary, impulsive, demanding, and concretist. They have stereotyped cognitive styles, and exploitative and dependent interpersonal styles" (Hauser et al., 1984, p. 196). During the later conformist stage, individuals develop the ability to express inner states verbally, and there is a "gradual increase in self-awareness and an appreciation of the multiple possibilities of a situation" (p. 196). In the most advanced stage of ego development, the postconformist stage, an individual is able to cope with inner conflict through a high degree of self-perception. Accompanied by complex cognitive skills and understanding, this level of ego development translates into an interpersonal style that emphasizes mutuality, autonomy, empathy, and acceptance of individual differences. Although these stages are not necessarily age related (adults and adolescents may range from the earliest to the latest phases), it is likely that more sophisticated ego development will occur with increasing age. Mutual and empathetic relationships, in which partners have more realistic perceptions of their status, increase their chances of avoiding negative consequences of their sexual conduct.

With growing identity formation and ego development, many aspects of teenagers' lives become more stable. The younger the adolescent, the less likely that a relationship will be long term, but also the more likely that it will be unrealistically perceived. Young people may be sure that a relationship will last into the future, despite overwhelming evidence that their lives are in constant flux. Counselors report that their inability to recognize the possibility of change leads adolescent girls to depend inordinately on the stability of a current relationship, however brief it is, despite previous experience of short, sequential partnerships.

On the one hand, the lack of long-term commitment is desirable at this stage; we would not want to see young adolescents locked into "stable" relationships. On the other hand, such lack of stability impedes protective behavior. It is likely to be associated with multiple partners, even if in the context of sequential monogamy. It is unlikely to be associated with the ability to communicate adequately with a partner. The use of contraception, particularly during early experiences of intercourse, when the condom is most likely to be the method available, requires a level of openness about the sexual reality of a relationship. There is clear evidence that the use of contraception is enhanced by high dyadic commitment, both because it improves communication between partners and because it makes it more likely that the young woman will acknowledge the probability that coitus will occur.

The quality of the relationship within which sex takes place is not perceived similarly by male and female teenagers. Young women desire stronger relationships with their partners before having intercourse than do young men. Similarly a young woman tends to describe the relationship with her last sexual partner as stronger than does a young man. Nearly 80% of female adolescents in a high school sample describe the relationship with the most recent partner as a strong one, compared with only 41% of males in the same sample (Zabin, Hirsch, Smith, & Hardy, 1984). Only 10% of the young women describe the relationship as weak, compared with 42% of the young men. This difference can have an important impact on the risks faced by these young women, who are less likely to seek contraception for sexual contact within a relationship that they do not think will last. As we will see, it is not the risk they run at each sexual encounter that finally drives them to seek protection, but the perception of an ongoing relationship in which they can express the expectation of future encounters.

The stages of sexual intimacy through which adolescents pass may be dissociated from the emotional intimacy they feel. The younger the teenagers are at first coitus, the more likely that it involves a minimal level of intimacy; at these ages, the incidence of casual sex is greatest and relationships are weakest. Also at these ages, the probability that sexual contact is involuntary is great (Moore et al., 1989); even when it cannot be characterized as "abuse," the level of emotional involvement is often minimal.

Stages of Intimacy

Early descriptions of adolescent sexuality delineated a progression of sexual behaviors, with physical contact increasing over a relatively long succession of stages before coitus (Bentler, 1968; Brady & Levitt, 1965; Sorenson, 1973; Spanier, 1975). Smith and Udry (1985) described noncoital sexual behaviors that range from kissing, through necking and petting above and below the waist, with and without clothes. It is generally assumed that adolescents pass through each stage in this sequence before engaging in intercourse. The importance of this sequence, however, varies among social groups. Evidence suggests that, among black adolescents, intercourse is often an earlier form of sexual expression than among whites and may precede some noncoital behaviors. In this group, experience of one stage of intimacy does not predict the future timing of the next stage, whereas among white adolescents, the progression is fairly predictable. For example, among white females, the chance of experiencing intercourse within 2 years is 50% for those who have engaged in unclothed petting; among white males, this same probability obtains among those who have participated in below-the-waist petting. Among black adolescents, however, there is no predictable progression of precoital activity. Among males and females, although precoital activity is also associated with a 50% chance of experiencing coitus within 2 years, more have experienced intercourse than unclothed petting.

This kind of information alerts the clinician to some important aspects of early adolescent sexual activity. The meaning of sexual intimacy, its role in relationships, and the evolution of sexual behaviors among adolescents are aspects of sexuality that have been neglected—perhaps because a desire to promote contraceptive behaviors has focused attention on the onset of intercourse as a marker of pregnancy risk (Brooks-Gunn & Furstenberg, 1989). But not all groups pass through the same stages of physical contact on the way to intercourse. If premature coitus cuts short or accelerates the progression of physical intimacy, the timing of pregnancy risk will come chronologically earlier even if male-female relationships are initiated at the same age. In turn, if intercourse plays a different role within different cultural groups, then interventions to decrease risky behavior, and the optimal timing of those interventions, must vary dramatically as well.

Planning for Intercourse

One of the mediating factors that links the strength of a relationship to contraceptive use is the expectation that coitus will take place. Whether or not coitus has taken place in the past or is likely to take place in the future, the conscious expectation that it *will* take place is an important precondition for contraceptive preparation. Planning intercourse is not common among adolescents; the younger they are, the less likely that intercourse will be anticipated. And the younger the teenager, the more likely that first intercourse will also be unprotected.

Only 17% of teenage females and 35% of teenage males claim that their first intercourse was planned in advance (Zelnik & Shah, 1983). Planning was, not surprisingly, associated with a stronger relationship, with contraceptive use, and with the use of more effective methods. An inability to predict and plan for sexual encounters reflects normal cognitive limitations of adolescents, who have only a beginning conception of *possibility* and a limited orientation to the future. An important cognitive change in adolescence is the development of abstract thinking. Piaget (1972) suggested that the conception of "possibility" begins at about 12 years of age and that there are cortical changes related to the emergence of these cognitive capacities without which the concept of possibility can have no meaning. Characterized by an ability to think abstractly with concepts not tied to actual or experienced objects, the "formal" stage of operational thinking gives the cognitive underpinning for an understanding of probabilistic events; without that understanding, such risks as conception or the transmission of disease must appear remote. Elkind (1975) elaborated Piaget's stages into phases of logical growth: The development of certain logical constructs precedes an understanding not only of possibility but also of probability. Numerical probabilities represent an elusive reality for many adults; for adolescents, the concept of *likelihood* is remote. This lack of cognitive understanding constrains the ability to evaluate and act on future contingencies.

Similarly, without a reliable concept of the abstract and the possible, adolescents have limited orientation to the future. Abstract thinking and a clearer sense of time are required to understand messages such as "pregnancy will affect your future." It is unlikely that young adolescents will absorb this as a message with specific relevance to them or their lives, even when they have been taught the basics of human biology. Piaget said that anticipation, a precondition for most protective behaviors, is the hallmark of operative thinking. Because adolescents have difficulty using present resources to deal with the future, when those whose sexual onset is early fail to foresee and plan for protection despite the fact that they "know better"—and despite a vague desire to be responsible—they are not "deficient" in their development. They are constrained by normal limits to their cognitive capacities.

Frequency of intercourse is also linked to the expectation that intercourse will take place. An expectation that intercourse is going to happen more frequently prompts some adolescents to obtain contraceptive counseling. Associated as it is with closer, more stable relationships, frequency may be a marker for the quality of the relationship. It may be that the *infrequency* of coitus in this age group does reduce the statistical risk to a cohort of adolescents, but it gives an individual teenager very little protection. Similarly the long periods of abstinence between monogamous relationships that most teenagers experience, although they may reduce exposure, may also serve to compound their risk: They may stop using whatever method they have adopted with the end of one relationship and then commence a new relationship without protection (Hirsch & Zelnik, 1985). Thus sporadic intercourse is not always the protective factor it might appear; it is often associated with increased, not decreased, risk.

Sexual Self-Image

That so many young women allow intercourse to "just happen," despite its profound implications for their future lives, is cause for concern. There are many reasons why a young woman may perceive this event as unplanned. Her surprise may reflect lack of desire for intercourse, which may be connected with some degree of coercion, physical or otherwise. However, she may also be denying any volition on her part in defense against her own half-formed moral structures, because she is not ready to accept her sexual identity by anticipating or planning intercourse. The development of a sexual self-image may be a prerequisite for engaging in the decision-making process that precedes contraceptive use. To undertake the necessary practical steps, from seeking health care and undergoing physical examination to taking, inserting, applying, or talking about contraception, requires some comfort with bodily aspects of sex, as well as with the idea of one's own sexuality.

A readiness to recognize the sexual self may offer a partial explanation for the importance of the quality of the relationship in encouraging contraceptive use. It appears to be the emotional quality of a relationship, rather than the fact of coital contact, that causes young women to recognize their need for protection. That a young woman does not anticipate intercourse may also indicate that her relationships are all either so intense or so casual that the concept of *stages of intimacy* has no real meaning for her; anticipating sexual intercourse may be difficult because the cues that could provide for anticipation are absent. Either for this reason or because it is not associated with intimacy, the act of intercourse may be psychologically separated from the closeness that most young women seek with their sexual partners.

The development of a sexual self-image is inevitably tied to age and to the normative environment in which the adolescent lives. But, although sexual behavior is surrounded by norms and taboos, there is nonetheless a personal factor in the equation. Thus, in an attempt to make personal choices, adolescents and adults alike enter the arena of moral deliberation. For the adolescent, however, that deliberation is constrained by the emerging struggle to develop a personal moral code. Kohlberg (1964) identified changes in moral reasoning during adolescence both with Piaget's cognitive stages and Eriksen's levels of identity formation. Although not all persons develop moral judgment equivalent to their cognitive capacity, he contended that they cannot develop it beyond that level. Thus cognitive development puts stringent limits on the moral reasoning of early adolescents, and changes in moral beliefs related to sexuality during the teen years are related to these evolving capacities. These changes occur during the same stressful period characterized by adolescents' increasing permissiveness as they separate from family and identify more and more with their peers.

The development of a personal moral code is a long process, even when it builds on the foundation of a mature self-image. It is small wonder that young adolescents, struggling with an immature sense of self and dependent on external reactions for self-definition, with only a dawning awareness of the nature of personal volition and self-control (Damon & Hart, 1982), are at high risk for unplanned, unprotective behavior in many areas of their lives. Nor is it unusual that they should display apparently contradictory, ambivalent, and so-called irresponsible behavior in their sexual lives. The cognitive capacity to understand the full implications of one's actions develops late and changes continuously throughout the teenage years. A few years' difference in the age at which particular behaviors are inaugurated can make a major difference in their management.

BARRIERS TO CONTRACEPTIVE USE

Why Adolescents Delay

In an attempt to understand what teenagers themselves feel are barriers to their utilization of professional contraceptive services, young women attending 32 family planning clinics nationwide for a first such visit were asked to reply to an anonymous questionnaire that probed their reasons for delay (Zabin & Clark, 1981). Table 4.1 presents their responses both

TABLE 4.1 Percentage Distribution of Respondents by Different Reasons Cited as Most Important for Delaying Their First Clinic Visit; and Percentage Citing Each Reason as Contributing to Their Delay

Reason	% Distribution by Most Important Reason (N=934)	% Citing as Contributing Reason (N=1,049)
Just didn't get around to it	15.0	38.1
Afraid my family would find out if I came	12.1	31.0
Waiting for closer relationship with partner	12.0	27.6
Afraid to be examined	8.5	24.8
Thought birth control dangerous	7.9	26.5
Never thought of it	6.9	16.4
Didn't think had sex often enough to get pregnant	3.6	16.5
Didn't know where to get birth control help	3.3	15.3
Didn't expect to have sex	3.3	12.8
Thought birth control I was using was good enough	3.1	7.8
Thought I was too young to get pregnant	2.8	11.5
Thought it cost too much	2.5	18.5
Partner opposed	2.5	8.4
Thought I had to be older to get birth control	2.1	13.1
Thought birth control wrong	1.1	9.2
Thought I wanted pregnancy	1.1	8.4
Forced to have sex	0.7	1.4
Sex with relative	0.1	0.7
Other	10.7	9.7
Total	100.0	na

NOTE: na = not applicable

to a query about *all* the reasons that contributed to their delay and to one that asked them to select the single most important reason. The answers cover many areas of concern. Some suggest a lack of information, others suggest fear, and still others reflect attitudes that are typically associated with the adolescent years. In a follow-up study using the same question some years later in a nonclinic, school population, the importance of the same reasons was confirmed (Zabin, Stark, & Emerson, 1991). In the sections that follow, several types of the teenagers' responses will be addressed as we examine personal and institutional barriers to protective behavior in this age group.

Knowledge and Perceptions
of Conception and Contraception

It is well understood that knowledge does not predict behavior. Early studies (Pool & Pool, 1978; Shah, Zelnik, & Kantner, 1975; Sorenson, 1973) found that some of the reasons given by adolescent women for their nonuse of contraceptives implied a basic lack of knowledge about the possibility of becoming pregnant. More recently, reviewers continue to conclude that teenagers have gaps in basic understanding of reproductive physiology (Brooks-Gunn & Furstenberg, 1989; Morrison, 1985). Morrison, in a comprehensive review of the psychology of contraceptive use in adolescence, concluded that there is still only a superficial and limited knowledge of basic reproductive facts and the various methods of contraception. This conclusion was drawn from research on reasons for nonuse of contraception, not from tests of intellectual knowledge. She found that "a sizable proportion of teenagers are uninformed about basic physiology . . . and believe that they are immune to pregnancy despite theoretical probability" (Morrison, 1985, p. 564).

Some reasons given by teenagers for not using contraception (Table 4.1), such as they had intercourse too infrequently, only once, or at the wrong time of month (when indeed they are ignorant of the ovulation cycle) or that they are too young to conceive, imply inadequate knowledge of the physiology of reproduction. We have found, however, that the same young women who give these responses often give accurate answers when asked the abstract facts of sex and pregnancy risk. Most of the young women who reported (well after their own menarche) that they thought they were "too young" to get pregnant knew that a girl can conceive immediately after menarche. Most of those whose reason for delay in obtaining contraception was that they did not have sex "often enough" knew that a woman could conceive after only one coital experience. The problem does not appear to be a lack of knowledge but an inability to internalize that knowledge, to apply it to their hazard rate, and to act on it. Lack of knowledge cannot explain sporadic or intermittent contraceptive use, but such use can be explained if nonuse does not reflect a lack of abstract information but an inability to translate it into action.

An understanding of sexual biology cannot be taken for granted simply because the facts have been imparted; there is evidence that this information demands a relatively high level of cognitive development before it is adequately comprehended, and without such a cognitive context, sexual information is transformed by children to fit their own cognitive levels (Bernstein & Cowan, 1975). This conclusion does not explain cross-cultural differences in understanding reproductive physiology; there is evidence that North American teenagers lag behind their European counterparts in comprehending "how babies are made," suggesting a cultural component (Goldman & Goldman, 1982). Among North American children at 13 years of age, 50% gave an overtly sexual explanation, whereas among Swedish children, a similar proportion gave such answers by 9 years of age.

Reasons for not using contraception are not confined to lack of awareness of birth control options or of the risk of pregnancy. They include a large measure of fear and misinformation about its use, as well as ambivalence about childbearing itself. Although levels of awareness about methods of contraception and their availability are generally high, teenagers' perceptions of the risks and benefits associated with its use are often extremely negative. Inaccurate beliefs about the dangers and ineffectiveness of contraception are sufficiently strong to discourage them from addressing the many problems associated with its acquisition and use. For example, teenagers have exaggerated fears about the side effects of the pill. In view of the fact that these perceptions are the most effective barriers to use among adult women in the United States (Silverman, Torres, & Forrest, 1987), it is not surprising that, among the adolescents in clinic and school samples, the belief that birth control is dangerous ranks consistently in the first five most frequently cited reasons for delaying a contraceptive visit (Zabin & Clark, 1981; Zabin, Stark, & Emerson, 1991). The longest delays between the initiation of intercourse and attendance at a family planning clinic are associated with the belief that the method the girl is already using is "good enough" and with a belief that contraception is "wrong." Beliefs that contraception is morally or medically objectionable have been shown to be most prevalent among people of low educational background and low socioeconomic status, but in all groups such beliefs are often another reflection of a general discomfort with sexual activity itself.

Negative beliefs and attitudes about contraception are not limited to matters of statistical effectiveness and danger. Adolescents share with adults feelings that contraception is uncomfortable, awkward, or unattractive. Sterilization is now the most widely used method of birth control among married adults in their 30s in the United States, presumably reflecting the fact that "they have many of the same apprehensions and problems with contraception that teenagers do" (Brooks-Gunn & Furstenberg, 1989, p. 253). This discomfort may manifest the generalized ambivalence and lack of realism about sex in American culture. An indefinable negativity led Morrison to conclude that "the failure to find specific negative attributes of contraception that are reliable across studies lends support to the hypothesis that some generalized negative affect toward sex-related topics is one component underlying adolescents' attitudes toward using contraceptives" (1985, p. 565).

Partner Relationships

Adolescent women are commonly "waiting for a closer relationship" with their partners before seeking contraceptive counseling (Table 4.1). Among white females, communication with the partner is associated with shorter delays in attending a clinic, although the relationship between communication and delay is not consistent among black females. The perception of "closeness," the communication that goes with it, and the mutual responsibility that characterizes a close relationship all enhance contraceptive use. Unfortunately, the younger the teenager, the less likely that their relationships will qualify as "close."

What is of interest about that response, shown in Table 4.1, is that it was given not by young women who had just initiated coitus but by young women who had often been involved in coital contact for more than a year (Zabin & Clark, 1981). What did they mean when they said they were awaiting a closer relationship? Surely they did not mean to suggest that one does not try to avoid pregnancy with a casual partner but only with one with whom the relationship is intimate. Rather it would seem that they implied the importance of a close relationship in permitting one to anticipate coitus. And, perhaps, the importance of a close relationship in permitting one to see oneself as a sexual being, for whom the act of seeking protection is legitimate and even appropriate.

Male partners' feelings about contraception, or rather young women's perceptions of their male partners' feelings, also interfere with the decision-making process; the younger the woman, the more likely she is to be swayed by her partner's perceived opinion. Complaints that a partner objects to the use of birth control, that contraception interferes with spontaneity or the pleasure of sex, inhibit the use of both male and female methods of contraception. These arguments may be seen as reflecting a functional lack of access to contraception at the moment of coitus or a psychological inability to accept the sexual role. The relationship between attachment and contraception is probably not only one of frequency and continuity but also one of intimacy. Goldsmith found that those whose mutual desire for coitus are strongest are most protected (Goldsmith, Gabrielson, Gabrielson, Matthews, 1972). Intimacy is central to communication and to the mutual assumption of responsibility to protect one another from the negative consequences of coitus.

Crisis Orientation

Many adolescents and adults have a crisis orientation to health care and thus to contraception. A high proportion of teenage women first attend a clinic for a pregnancy test, attesting to the importance of specific events provoking a crisis immediate enough to stimulate action. Those young women who are least crisis oriented and seek contraceptive advice in anticipation of first intercourse are most likely to recognize their personal risk, whereas an internalization of risk is lowest among those who first come to a clinic for a pregnancy test (Zabin & Clark, 1981).

The experience of a pregnancy test does not necessarily lead a young woman to a more realistic appraisal of her own vulnerability—a consequence often assumed to result from a pregnancy "scare." Young women who experience negative tests are in fact at high risk of a future unintended pregnancy (Zabin, Hirsch, & Boscia, 1990; Zabin et al., 1989). Their continued risk of conceiving reflects not only their considerable ambivalence about a potential pregnancy but for some probably represents the effects of the adolescent fable of invulnerability.

Lack of planning is also reflected in the fact that only 14% of adolescents attending an urban family planning clinic for the first time came as virgins, in anticipation of first intercourse (Zabin & Clark, 1981). Over 36% came only after they suspected that they were pregnant. Among the others, the mean delay between first intercourse and clinic attendance was more than 16 months; the median was one year. Those who presented most promptly were most likely to have used a method before, a finding that indicates they had already evidenced some degree of preparedness. Nonprescription methods, which require preparation but not the forethought and commitment required for prescription methods, are an important source of protection for those who take control early; their use is associated with earlier, not later, use of effective medical methods.

Privacy

An important task of adolescence is the achievement of independence while still living at home with parents. It is often difficult for parents to see their offspring turn to peers rather than themselves as role models and counselors. But these are years of growing independence, even if a teenager's standards are firmly rooted in the home. Privacy becomes an essential part of this process, particularly in the realm of sexual behavior. Therefore confidentiality is the sine qua non of teen services. Adolescents are not only sensitive about privacy from parents. They turn to their peers for self-affirmation and hesitate to explain themselves or their motives to adults. Thus young boys are often embarrassed to ask an unfamiliar salesperson for condoms: An "imaginary audience" is watching them, and they don't want to give themselves away.

Thus, however ineffective the fear of parental disapproval is in preventing the occurrence of intercourse, it is very effective in preventing youngsters from protective behavior. "Fear that my family will find out" is consistently in the top three reasons for not having attended a clinic soon after sexual onset. This is a particularly cogent barrier for young white adolescents. If it is difficult for parents, it is for adolescents as well; their need to rely on parents while working on separation is not an easy task.

Procrastination

Many adolescents have far fewer concrete reasons for their contraceptive behavior. In clinic populations, 37.3% of the black sexually active teenage women said that "just not getting around to it" contributed to their delay in getting contraceptive services (Zabin & Clark, 1981), a response that was apparently just as frequent among whites. Nearly 14% of these women said that this was the most important reason for the interval between initiation of intercourse and seeking clinic attendance. These young women are acting like normal adolescents: Procrastination is not confined to any particular adolescent population, nor is it limited to sexual matters. To those who know teens, it is a familiar syndrome. Most teenagers need a level of reinforcement to achieve even mundane tasks that present none of the ambivalence and potential conflict associated with the use of contraception. They live in the present and are not easily motivated to act now for future goals. Their feelings of personal effectiveness are weak and often cause them to waver even about straightforward decisions.

Ambivalence and lack of openness surrounding sexuality compound their difficulty in acting on the need and desire for contraception. Ambivalence intensifies procrastination. Young teenagers' own moral uncertainty, as they both question and internalize external standards of behavior, is exacerbated by the contradictory messages they receive from the cultural milieu. On the one hand, sex (particularly between the young and beautiful) is glorified and exploited in the media. On the other hand, there is still societal disapproval of unwed parenthood, particularly teenage motherhood, in most social settings. Between these two messages there is almost no acknowledgement of contraception and an absence of realistic portrayals of sexual negotiation. It is not surprising that adolescents are often bewildered in the vacuum of information and advice about how to link the contradictory norms that surround them.

Practical Barriers

Functional barriers to clinic access certainly influence clinic utilization by teenagers; for young adolescents, the difficulty of negotiating the health care system is substantial. Practical processes such as scheduling appointments, finding transportation, maintaining secrecy, undergoing examination and interview, getting and paying for contraceptives, and then using them regularly and effectively are all beyond the capacity of many young teens. We have found that black teenagers often seek out contraceptive advice from clinics more promptly than white adolescents, perhaps reflecting their frequent contact with a clinical setting that can provide continuity of care. Among white adolescents, who because of their socioeconomic status are more likely to have no such affiliation, the age of 16 seems to form a threshold at which, regardless of age at first intercourse, they feel able to find and attend a clinic.

Recent work indicates that although cost and physical barriers are important to some young women, the barriers imposed by their attitudes and perceptions are at least as important. Although this does not negate the need for free, convenient, confidential services, it suggests the need for compassionate and appropriate care as well. The clinic experience, the attitudes of health care providers and counselors, and the ease with which the adolescent feels she can receive attention will either intensify or counter the ambivalence, procrastination, functional difficulty, and even fear that can underlie the nonuse of contraception.

ATTITUDES AND BEHAVIOR

Early initiation of coitus and a lack of contraceptive use are often seen as evidence of irresponsible attitudes toward moral behavior among the current generation of youth. But, on the contrary, when teenagers are given the chance to express their attitudes anonymously, they generally report attitudes that are quite consistent with responsible sexual behavior (Zabin, Hirsch, et al., 1984). Not unlike many of their adult role models, they frequently experience difficulty translating their beliefs into conduct.

Among a sample of sexually experienced urban adolescents, 83% gave a "best" age for first intercourse that was older than the age at which they themselves had experienced that event; in fact, 43% cited an age older than their *current* age. Similarly, among young mothers in the sample, 88% said that the best age to have a baby is older than the age at which they had borne a child. Among both sexually active and virgin adolescents, 39% of females and 32% of males believed that premarital sex is wrong. This proportion was much higher among virgins, but 25% of those who had already had intercourse shared this view (Zabin, Hirsch, et al., 1984).

Attitudes about contraceptive responsibility are statistically associated with contraceptive use, as might be expected, but for a sizeable number of respondents to the same survey, the attitude and the behavior were discrepant. Those adolescents who considered it the responsibility of both partners to prevent pregnancy were most likely to have used some method of contraception at last intercourse, followed by those who saw this responsibility as belonging to only one or other of the partners. Those who believed that pregnancy prevention is not the responsibility of either partner were the least likely to have used a method of contraception at last intercourse. Nevertheless, of those who assigned responsibility to one or both partners, 32% of women and 37% of men used no protection at last intercourse. Of those who answered "true" to the statement "I would only have sex if one of us was using some kind of birth control," 21% of females and 26% of males had not used a method at last coitus.

The reasons for such incongruence of belief and action are probably many, although the phenomenon is hardly unusual. In the context of adolescent psychological development, two factors may be relevant. First, adolescent responses to "what is ideal" may be triggered by the normative pressures of the social context. Family, friends, community, and media have an impact on young people's perception of ideal and right behaviors, even though these perceived norms may not translate into a personal code of conduct. Or the responses may represent the adolescents' perception of what ought to be, while their actions reflect the norms around them. The stated attitudes and actual behaviors of young women are more consistent than those of young men. This difference may reflect a greater need among the teenage women to believe that their behavior is consistent with generalized norms because they are under more social control; deviance, its perceived value and implications, may well be different for them than for males. Second, adolescents themselves may not be aware of the inconsistencies in their answers. In light of the disparate nature of self-understanding in adolescence and the incomplete process of internalizing external norms, differences between the ideal and the actual may not concern them.

The nature of the causal relationship between attitude and behavior is debatable. Behavioral change may precede attitudinal change, or attitudes may change behavior. The pace of change in adolescents' self-perception and the meaning of the social self may be reflected in constantly shifting sexual attitudes and in behaviors often out of alignment with beliefs. Or teenagers may not be happy about experiences they have had; attitudinal responses may represent an attempt to advocate for a different norm. For example, differences between ideal and actual ages of intercourse or childbearing, particularly after the event, may indicate regret, misgiving, or the wish that they had had more control over those events.

For interventions that try to change teenagers' risk-taking behavior, the disparity between attitudes and behavior implies that neither intellectual knowledge nor responsible attitudes may translate into congruent actions. The process of internalization is complex and long, and sexual behavior, even among adults, is replete with tensions between the desired and the actual.

CONCLUSION

The age at which a young person engages in sexual contact has a profound effect on the way these behaviors are managed and understood. Too often, in adolescence, they put the young person at risk emotionally, physically, and in terms of his or her future development and future goals. Some risk factors derive from the social settings in which early onset is likely to occur but nonetheless compound the problem. Age is no guarantee of protective behavior, but in early adolescence the risks are great.

Under certain conditions, an adolescent is likely to be protected from unwanted pregnancy and sexually transmitted diseases: These are generally situations in which the young woman is in a stable relationship, can communicate with her partner, and shares with him a responsibility to prevent pregnancy. Such relationships are probably longer in duration and occasion more frequent and predictable episodes of intercourse. Teenagers probably benefit from others' perception of them as sexual beings, facilitating their own acceptance of that role. Protection is enhanced when young people have internalized their personal risk, acknowledging their susceptibility to disease and pregnancy. All these conditions are most likely to obtain in the later teenage years. Such conditions as a stable relationship, a realistic perception of risk, and an adequate sexual self-image are precluded by the developmental stage of the adolescent when onset is early. Therefore only interventions that respond to the developmental status of the adolescent are able to give her the protection she requires.

5

CHILDBEARING: ITS CONSEQUENCES AND MANAGEMENT

INTRODUCTION

Although unintended childbearing is one of the most obvious consequences of youthful sexual activity, we address it separately because it
is a quite different manifestation of that activity from those considered
in the previous chapter. Not only does childbearing involve another life,
but it also is experienced by a restricted subset of sexually active youth.
Issues relating to the nature of adolescent partnerships, to the use and
nonuse of contraception, to sexually transmitted diseases, and even to
the decision to terminate or carry an unwanted conception are of
concern in all social and economic groups in the United States. Adolescent childbearing, on the other hand, has become almost normative only
in areas of economic deprivation. In turn, the problems we see that
relate to early childbearing—problems of prenatal care, single parenthood, economic dependency, and immature parenting, for example—
are frequently related not only to the adolescent's child but to the
underlying poverty into which the child is born.

In this chapter, we will discuss briefly some of the social and economic consequences of childbearing during the adolescent years in
order to explore the direction of causality and to separate as well as we
can those outcomes that are probably sequelae of the circumstances in
which the child was conceived and those that appear to be independent
effects of childbearing. We will examine the reasons that may underlie
the decision to bear a child and the relationships between those reasons
and the social setting of the young mother. We will then address the

nature of the medical problems associated with the management of adolescents' pregnancies and finally the consequences to the children of adolescent mothers.

CONSEQUENCES OF EARLY PARENTHOOD

For many years, the literature stressed the problem of poor educational attainment among young mothers compared with later childbearing peers. Even when secular improvements were noted among mothers, they were generally smaller than increments in the same period experienced by females who had not borne children in adolescence. These deficits were confirmed when prior achievement and aspirations were controlled (Card & Wise, 1978; Hayes, 1987). More recent literature based on event histories demonstrates that periods of chronic absence from school generally predate the conception or birth of a child (Upchurch & McCarthy, 1990), suggesting that low achievement is in a causal relationship with both school dropout and childbearing. The child rarely interrupts an intact educational career. A poor rate of return following the birth of a child, however, confirms the fact that childbearing makes an independent contribution to high school completion, which not surprisingly is associated with more economic dependency in the subsequent years. That relationship, in turn, has been well documented; some of its manifestations are discussed elsewhere in this chapter, as well as in Chapter 2, and need not be detailed here.

Single parenthood (see Chapter 2) and insecure partnerships are also more common among those who become parents in adolescence. Fathers of babies born to teenagers, whether or not they are teenagers themselves, are likely to be poorly educated and dependent on their own families, a situation that increases the probability that their children will live in deprived and transient circumstances.

Dependency is likely to increase not only for the young mother but also for her primary family if she and her child remain with them, as is frequently the case, especially within the black community. Whether dependency is measured by welfare receipt or by a ratio of working adults to the total number of persons in the household, there is evidence of an increase in dependency during the year or two following the birth, relative to a like period among those who do not bear a child (Zabin, Wong, Weinick, & Emerson, 1992).

In this context, both the nature and strength of the family support system can have an important influence on the developmental course of a young person (Boyce, Schaeffer, & Uitti, 1985). In their longitudinal study of mothers who bore children by the age of 17, Furstenberg et al. found that family support was a key factor in ameliorating the long-term negative effects of parenthood on the life of the adolescent mother herself (Furstenberg, 1976; Furstenberg & Brooks-Gunn, 1987). It is the financial and child care support of the primary family that makes it possible for the young mother to return to school; this support is more likely to be given by a black family than a white family, hence the higher probability that a young black mother completes her high school education.

Each of the consequences we have outlined, as well as those for the child, is intensified when the original birth is followed by others within the teen years. Medical sequelae for mother and child and outcomes for the children are addressed below.

WHY DO ADOLESCENTS BEAR CHILDREN?

Discussing a rationale for early parenthood does not imply that bearing a child, for most adolescents, is a reasoned process—a deliberate attempt to meet some need or to accomplish some objective. Indeed even young women who decide to carry their children rarely have conceived on purpose. In most studies, well over 80% of those who conceive say that the pregnancy was unintended (Hayes, 1987). In a study of girls age 17 and younger awaiting the results of their pregnancy tests, fewer than 5% of those who then carried their pregnancies said that they had wanted to conceive (Zabin et al., 1989).

Why do they not opt for abortion? The reasons appear to be very personal and specific to the pregnancy, not necessarily an opposition to abortion in general. In the same study, the differences in objective attitude toward abortion were minimal between those who terminated and those who carried (Zabin et al., 1990). All the young women, however, expressed considerable ambivalence in their answers to several questions that tapped their feelings about childbearing. Although few said that they "wanted" a child, many more said that they would be happy if they found out they had conceived or that a child would be no problem to them. In turn, there is a very strong relationship between ambivalence and childbearing; surprisingly, that association is just as strong as the relationship between wanting to conceive and bearing a child. The only group in the study with a significantly lower probability of childbearing consisted of those who consistently and unequivocally did not want to become pregnant: those who would be unhappy if it happened, who would find a child a problem, and who said they did not wish to conceive.

Ambivalence suggests not only that there have been multiple influences on the adolescent but also that there is no overriding reason to avoid childbearing. In light of the pressures on young people to initiate coitus described in Chapter 3 and the difficulties they experience in managing their sexual lives discussed in Chapter 4, it is hardly surprising that many conceive. Having conceived, those with a strong vision of a future with which a child would compete or those whose social setting assigns too high a cost to childbearing will generally opt for abortion. If those conditions do not apply, there will appear to be few reasons for the teenager *not* to bear her child, even if the rewards for so doing are also small. Thus, to the extent that adolescents foresee few benefits in their futures, an unintended birth carries few perceived costs. That assessment, while personal, is deeply affected by the family, the environment, and the peer setting.

The recent work of Horwitz and colleagues (Horwitz, Klerman, Kuo, & Jekel, 1991) gives some insight into one role that familial factors may play in the risk of teenage childbearing. In a recent long-term follow-up of young mothers from the late 1960s in New Haven, they found that among the offspring of these women, most had not become parents by the time they were 19 years old. Those who did become teenage parents were most likely to be female and to report significant depressive symptoms. They found that both male and female teenage parents were more likely to be the children of women who had moved out of their own mothers' homes within 26 months of the child's birth and to have suffered a lifetime of depression. They postulated that these factors imply a degree of emotional deprivation for the offspring most at risk, both due to the removal at an early age of a significant emotional figure and caregiver, the child's grandmother, as well as the emotional unavailability that is evident in the presence of depression. Such deprivation may lead adolescents to seek emotional closeness at an early age through sexual activity and having a child (Horwitz et al., 1991).

The impact of emotional isolation is confirmed in interviews with adolescent mothers (Boxill, 1987; Frank, 1983). Boxill reported that two of four major themes in adolescent mothers' experience concern their feelings of emotional poverty: first, they perceive failures in their own parents and an inability to communicate with them; second, they feel a lack of satisfactory relationships with peers and difficulty in establishing close relationships.

These explanations accord with early literature on out-of-wedlock childbearing in settings where it was relatively aberrational; in more recent literature, psychological explanations have tended to yield to others: It is suggested that premature parenthood may be part of a cluster of deviant—or at least detrimental—behaviors or that it may represent a transition to adulthood for those for whom alternative means of making that transition are lacking. Most convincing are contextual or environmental explanations for adolescent childbearing, which may in fact include aspects of each of the other descriptions, especially in communities where early, single parenthood has become almost normative.

As noted in Chapter 3, Hogan and Kitagawa (1985) found that residence in a ghetto neighborhood increased the risk of a pregnancy; this factor may operate through its impact on the family or independently. The assumption that a lack of opportunity or hope for the future is an important determinant of adolescent pregnancy is questioned by Jones and her colleagues (Jones, Forrest, Goldman, & Henshaw, 1985), who found teenagers' years of education and unemployment rates in European countries not significantly different from those in the United States—yet even in the presence of early sexual onset, childbearing is minimal. This argument, however, is based on national rates overall; it does not consider the educational and economic circumstances of inner-city urban populations in the United States. It may not take into account the European context, in which more varied educational and training options exist after age 16; because opportunities for various levels of qualification have considerable currency in the job market, traditional school education after that age is not considered to be an economic necessity. Nor does this analysis take into account feelings of racial oppression, which are very real to young people in the American ghetto setting (Boxill, 1987; Frank, 1983).

There is considerable interest in the pattern of intergenerational early and single motherhood. How the messages of the parent communicate to a child and the effects of parental communication on adolescent childbearing are not well understood. It seems clear that much of the communication is nonverbal; that is, the young person is well aware of parental attitudes toward childbearing and parenthood well before, and in the absence of, any direct communication on the subject. Perhaps the most powerful link between a mother's adolescent childbearing and that of her daughter is their shared environment. Similarly, associations between the behaviors of young women and their siblings, which exist but are not strong, are probably based on contextual factors.

THE PREGNANT ADOLESCENT AND HER CHILD

Are the children born to adolescents at higher risk? If so, are these risks medical, psychosocial, or economic in origin? From what do they derive, and can the management of the pregnancy in the antenatal and postnatal periods mitigate those risks in any way?

Regardless of age, maternal health prior to and during pregnancy affects the quality of the intrauterine environment and influences fetal development. Maternal malnutrition, illness, substance abuse, and infectious disease (particularly sexually transmitted disease) can have direct effects on the condition of the fetus and thus can influence its subsequent development. Although adolescence is often seen as a healthy time of life, young adolescents are in a transitional and demanding stage of growth and thus at risk of deficits in nutrition and health. These risks are compounded in just those settings where their likelihood of conceiving is high. The stress of pregnancy puts additional demands on the bodies of very young women that they may not be able optimally to meet. Consequently the growing fetus is more likely to be deprived, which can lead to a higher risk of intrauterine growth retardation and low birth weight (Institute of Medicine, 1985).

Intrauterine conditions are obviously not the only health determinants mediated through the mother. The cultural milieu mediates behaviors that can offset the detrimental effects of genetic or maternal conditions. Health beliefs and patterns of health care behavior are integral to any culture. Thus the perceived value of prenatal care, immunization, well-baby checkups, and such will determine in part the health-seeking behaviors that impact on the health and development of a child (Brown, 1989).

The Pregnant Adolescent

It would appear that, although from the biological point of view ages 18 and 19 are optimal childbearing years, during early adolescence there is an increased risk of low birth weight and perinatal mortality (Strobino, 1987). This risk has variously been pegged at 16 or 17 years and under. What is not as clear is the extent to which that excess risk is socioeconomic in origin, however real its physical manifestations. It is mediated in large measure by prenatal care. But the availability of good antenatal care and its utilization early in pregnancy are both related to such characteristics as low income, nonwhite race, unmarried status, low educational levels, and poor neighborhoods (Hardy & Zabin, 1991; Singh et al., 1985), all of which are also characteristics of most adolescents who bear children.

Other characteristics related to low birth weight are also frequently observed among adolescents. Infant size is related to prepregnancy weight of the mother, and many young mothers are small. Although maternal weight gain is often large for adolescents, nutrition may be poor, and the nutritional needs of young women during these years are greater than those of adult women. They may be competing with the fetus for nutrients that are in short supply either because of their socioeconomic status or their eating habits. Even when they consume more than enough calories, they may be deficient in certain vitamins, iron, and calcium. Iron can help prevent their increased risk of anemia, and calcium is indicated in the prevention of preeclampsia (toxemia of pregnancy), to which adolescents are particularly prone (Hardy & Zabin, 1991). The fact that they are biologically mature enough to carry does not imply that they have reached full growth; it may be that small size rather than their need for continued growth puts their infants at risk. Whatever its etiology, that risk is real.

Because of the clustering of high-risk behaviors described in Chapter 3, it is all too likely that the young mother will smoke or use drugs or alcohol. The relationship between drug use and low infant weight among teenage mothers has not been well established, but the danger to the infant of each of these behaviors is well documented. It may be that smoking explains much of the differential in outcomes among adolescents, as it does for adults. Negative sequelae among marijuana users are documented among adolescents and adults alike (McAnarney, 1987). Yet another confounding factor in the medical outcomes to adolescents is the presence of genital infection. Youthful sexual onset is often associated with multiple sexual partners and low socioeconomic status, both of which are risk factors for sexually transmitted disease; STDs in turn are risk factors for low birth weight and low gestational age.

Prenatal Care

It is very clear in the literature, whatever the source of excess risk, that an optimal level of care for young pregnant adolescents is crucial. With that level of care, negative outcomes have been reduced so that they compare favorably with adult outcomes; without that level of care, outcomes are consistently worse than those observed at older ages. This is particularly evident among multiparous adolescents whose babies are at increased risk with each pregnancy (Hardy & Zabin, 1991; McAnarney, 1987).

What are the aspects of high-risk care that have a documented association with improved outcomes? They include more frequent visits, nutritional counseling and supplementation, social work support for the adolescent mother and often for her family, and consistent care by providers who can serve as a bridge between regular prenatal care, auxiliary services, and delivery. The best success has been reported where case management systems have been utilized to integrate the skills of diverse service providers (Hardy & Zabin, 1991). The professionals who seem to maximize patient outcomes include counselors, health educators, and social workers whose services often cost considerably less than medical practitioners'; nonetheless, they are frequently dispensed with in medical settings when economic pressures are great. Thus an attempt to save money often produces negative sequelae that result in unacceptable human and financial costs. There is good evidence that many of those costs could be averted.

Children of Adolescents

It has been pointed out frequently that the characteristics of the normal teenager are in many ways the antithesis of those required for adequate parenting. The egocentrism and narcissism of youth are in sharp contrast to the mutuality that is required between mother and child or to the empathy that a young mother ideally will demonstrate with her offspring (Sadler & Catrone, 1983). Similarly, while the adolescent is struggling for independence from her family, her position within the family is changing; she often becomes more, not less, dependent on them for assistance and support. Still in the cognitive transition from concrete to formal operations, she is called on to solve problems beyond her capacities and to plan for the future for herself and her child. And, while still experimenting with roles of her own, she has to define for herself the difficult role of mother.

It is not surprising then that even when young mothers overcome many of the deficits of early parenthood and catch up with their peers in their educational and economic careers, the children demonstrate deficits of their own (Furstenberg & Brooks-Gunn, 1987). These deficits are documented in the area of personality and adjustment, behavior, and educational achievement; they extend to sexual conduct and early, unintended fertility. Although there is little evidence that neglect and abuse are specific to young mothers, associations between early motherhood and adverse sequelae, including criminal activity, are established in local and national samples.

Educational disadvantage starts young and often intensifies, although changes in the life course of the mother can have positive effects. We saw above that a solid maternal relationship can act as a protective factor against internal and external stressors; the practical and moral support offered across generations can counteract many of the adverse consequences of early childbearing on the life of the young mother (Furstenberg & Brooks-Gunn, 1987). But the intergenerational impact of major life events is hard to overcome. Although the mothers' and children's life trajectories intersect, and although the life course of the young mothers varies considerably and shows an enduring capacity for upward mobility even after years of public dependency, the children of these mothers experience negative effects. Even when deficits in the lives of the mothers were ameliorated, the stress of the early years is often passed on to the next generation. This evidence reinforces the importance of the environment in the early years of life; the negative impact of an adverse environment can be self-perpetuating.

Why do the children of these single, adolescent mothers exhibit the problems they do? First, as suggested above, the high-risk nature of the pregnancy itself can lead to poor outcomes such as intrauterine growth retardation, prematurity, and low birth weight, which may put children at early biological risk. It is often difficult to separate matters of biology and health from other mediating factors. The sequelae of illness may be offset by early intervention or exacerbated by a lack of resources, appropriate services, or the knowledge necessary to find them. The interaction of biology and environment is confirmed in the classic studies of Drillien (1964) and Werner and Smith (1982; Werner, 1985), who showed how protective factors such as innate characteristics of the child or mediating elements in the environment—including resources, family, and so on—can offset the adverse effects of biological or other stressors. Werner (1985) suggested that the more numerous the stressors, the more numerous and powerful must the protective factors be to offset them, a hypothesis similar to the model drawn by Jessor (1992) to explain the etiology of risk behavior. Protective factors may be in short supply in deprived and disorganized environments.

Specific family characteristics that influence the developmental course of a child include family structure, family environment, and family supports. Parental figures are central to children's security and sense of self. For optimal development, they require a close and stable affectional relationship with a parent, preferably two parents or a parent and grandmother, as well as interaction with other caring adults (Kellam, Adams, Brown, et al., 1982; Kellam, Ensminger, & Turner, 1977; McLanahan, 1983, 1985). Such relationships facilitate development and protect children living in adverse circumstances (Werner, 1985, 1986). It is difficult for the most committed and resourceful of parents to provide a favorable family environment in settings of poverty and social disruption. An atmosphere of well-being and order within the family enhances development even in the presence of economic deprivation. But that requires other resources, emotional and informational, rarely available to the adolescent. For young, single parents in areas where community and family resources are minimal, the odds against optimum parenting are therefore overwhelming.

In contrast to the optimal family setting, we have shown the considerable level of transiency that is evident in households of young inner-city mothers and their children (Zabin, Wong, et al., 1992). Furstenberg and Brooks-Gunn (1987) have shown the transient living arrangements that continue through the children's adolescence. Although an extended family can often provide surrogate parents who help support the child emotionally and economically, all too frequently it also provides a constant flow into and out of the family circle. The effect of this transiency on the young child is an area that requires study. Our own work has also shown that the economic well-being of the family in the years following the birth of a child to an adolescent is highly dependent on the ability of the young mother herself to enter the work force (Zabin, Wong, et al., 1992). Many young mothers are unable to do this, and the household increases in dependency. Others do so and at the same time attend school; thus they assist their families in the short run and improve their own opportunities in the long run. But their children apparently pay the price for the catch-up process. As biological and environmental pressures interact, sometimes ameliorating, sometimes exacerbating the effects of one another, two processes are occurring simultaneously;

one is horizontal, the other longitudinal. Although the influences of individual biology and social environment interact in a horizontal fashion, intergenerationally, genetics, parental behavior, and culture impact on the child. Whcn an intergenerational pattern of early childbearing is observed, both longitudinal and horizontal influences have had their effects. Within the brief span of 15 years or less, the same conditions that made the mother a child may make it much more likely that the vulnerable female child will become a mother.

CONCLUSION

It is difficult to separate the adverse consequences of childbearing in adolescence from the effects of the environments in which this pattern of parenting frequently occurs. There is evidence of independent educational and economic effects, over and above those characteristics of the young girl that put her at risk of early motherhood. The ability of many young women to "catch-up" with their peers who did not bear children during their teen years is impressive. However, it would appear that their children are in double jeopardy, biological and environmental, and do not fare as well. When the conditions for their development are mediated by the maternal behavior of an adolescent, influenced by the culture and circumstances that prevail in disadvantaged settings, the child may be especially vulnerable. A generation in some of our most disadvantaged neighborhoods may be of fewer than 15 years' duration; if the effects of early parenthood for mother and child are not addressed, they will reappear in a few short years in the children of the babies born today.

6

INTERVENTIONS

INTRODUCTION

The comprehensive model of sexual onset we described in Chapter 3, a model also relevant to adolescent childbearing, suggests a question crucial to intervention: Does such a model imply that the environment in which a young woman is reared and the developmental events that precede first intercourse are so powerful that they predetermine the outcome of her sexual decision making once she has an opportunity to initiate intercourse? Is a young man set on a course that predetermines the sexual roles he will play? If so, the possibilities for intervention would be extremely limited.

Many service providers believe in the importance of self-esteem in mediating the risk of pregnancy; that belief implies that the adolescent retains the power to make critical decisions whatever the historical influence of his or her environment. It implies that an intervention that changes adolescents' perceptions of themselves and their aspirations and expectations for the future can change the calculus of choice in any social setting. Similarly, one would then assume that educational programs that improve the knowledge on which adolescents base their decisions or service programs that make the means to manage those decisions available to them could also have a positive effect. If that is true, if it is possible for an intervention to change the choices that adolescents make at each step of the decision-making process, programs that work with individual adolescents may make an important difference in their lives.

However, the setting in which decisions are made with respect to early sexual relationships, unplanned pregnancy, and teenage parenthood is often far more powerful than any intervention that serves individual clients or patients. No single program can hope to combat the media messages that bombard young people at every socioeconomic level or the peer pressures and partner pressures that surround them. Providers who work with disadvantaged youth are well aware that poverty, unemployment, inadequate education, second-rate health care, and family stress also defy individual prescription. Such providers are rarely in a position to redress these problems; the help they give their clients can rarely change the personal, economic, or social circumstances of their lives. One may hope that society will eventually address the deep-rooted social malaise that underlies high rates of unwanted conception and pregnancy among the young, but this belief ought not delay our attempts to intervene.

Teenage pregnancy is not a new issue; it has been on the nation's reproductive health agenda for two decades (Hayes, 1987; Nathanson, 1991). Numerous interventions have been tried and documented. Even though many creative initiatives have never been well evaluated, we have learned enough for policymakers, planners, and providers to take constructive steps. A number of interventions have demonstrated measurable impact on rates of sexual activity and adolescent pregnancy and have led one analyst to conclude that it is a lack of political will, not a lack of knowledge, that prevents the implementation of effective programs, programs designed not so much to "beat the odds" as to change them (Schorr, 1985).

With a phenomenon as multifaceted as adolescent pregnancy, effective interventions cannot be neatly categorized by the particular helping profession that delivers the service, the service delivery setting, or the type of service that is offered. Programs that have the potential to reduce the incidence of adolescent sexual onset, pregnancy, and childbearing can intervene on many levels, in many settings, and at many points in the trajectory that leads to very early parenthood. Teenagers may encounter service providers before they have engaged in sexual intercourse, soon after first coitus, or after months or years of sexual activity; before conception, when they suspect a pregnancy or when one has been confirmed; before they decide which outcome to choose for a particular pregnancy, before an induced abortion or after it; during prenatal care, the postpartum period, or during early months of parenting. At each stage, there is an opportunity to intervene with education, counseling, and medical care. Intervention may belong most appropriately with a teacher, social worker, health educator, counselor, or psychologist; a nurse, nurse practitioner, or midwife; a pediatrician, family doctor, internist, obstetrician, or psychiatrist. Even those whom the adolescent first encounters—the receptionists, telephone operators, volunteers, and nursing aids who greet her—can be important links in the chain of effective intervention.

Nor can services be categorized by the needs of the young clients; even adolescents with similar problems may require very different levels of care. Services necessary for one individual may not be for another; services effective for one may be insufficient for another. Our research has shown that in many cases relationships of trust and understanding are at the beginning of behavior change and provide the key that helps some young people establish control over their lives. Although the life course of a young person can be changed by timely interaction with a sensitive and well-trained adult, youth who are most at risk may be inaccessible to the service community. They are often the most difficult to reach. For example, with the high drop-out rates that obtain in urban schools, services delivered through the schools—in programs conceived to *increase* accessibility—will miss large proportions of those most in need. Therefore every opportunity must be taken to address the needs of teenagers fully at whatever point they first make contact with the health or education delivery system; they may not be accessible again if that moment is lost.

CATEGORIES OF INTERVENTION

Preventive interventions aimed at helping young people avoid unwanted pregnancies and parenthood have commonly been divided into three general categories: educational programs, reproductive health programs, and a broad category often referred to as "life options" programs (Dryfoos, 1983; Hayes, 1987).

Educational Interventions

These programs are designed to increase levels of knowledge about human sexuality, sexually transmitted diseases, conception, contraception, pregnancy, and parenthood. Education also seeks to enhance the ability of young people to make responsible decisions about their sexuality by supporting or influencing their personal values and by affecting their social perceptions, attitudes, and skills. Programs that address this goal are usually but not always implemented through schools and include sex education and family life education. A variety of more innovative approaches has developed with this goal in mind: Assertiveness and decision-making training, family communication programs, teenage theater projects, and mass media initiatives are all being tried.

Evaluation of educational interventions has generally been limited to traditional or didactic sex education; it frequently measures success by changes in levels of knowledge—the explicit objective of most of these programs. It is clear that education does generally achieve this goal, especially among younger teens (Kirby, 1984). It has been reported that these interventions can also have a measurable effect on contraceptive use (Dawson, 1986; Marsiglio & Mott, 1986). By itself, information rarely has an impact on rates of sexual activity or pregnancy. However, recent advances in educational methods based on new models of behavior change (e.g., the health belief model, the social influence model, and social learning theory) have demonstrated some success in postponing sexual onset and in improving contraceptive practice (Eisen, Zellman, & McAlister, 1990; Howard & McCabe, 1990; Kirby, Barth, Leland, & Fetro, 1991). The same intervention will not necessarily meet the needs of all young people; such programs appear to have a greater impact on some subgroups than others. The behaviors of those who are not sexually active are more likely to be influenced (Danielson, Marcy, Plunkett, Weist, & Greenlick, 1990; Eisen et al., 1990; Howard & McCabe, 1990; Kirby, Barth, et al., 1991); some programs have more success with males than females (Eisen et al., 1990). Educational interventions are more likely to demonstrate behavior change when they are associated with medical intervention and counseling.

Although more is needed, education is the beginning of effective intervention. Moreover there is increasing approval for the inclusion of sex education in school curricula; more than four out of five parents favor it, and a majority favor services delivered through the schools as well. In light of this level of support and the primary role that knowledge can play in risk reduction, it is unfortunate that those who teach sex education in the United States so often feel that they are under pressure from school authorities and/or parents (Forrest & Silverman, 1989). Teachers also report a lack of training and materials to carry out their work. Furthermore, education in this field is frequently superficial and often omits important areas of information that adolescents require. Although fear of AIDS has prompted increased acceptance of sex education, pregnancy prevention receives far less attention than other risks of sexual activity (Rosoff, 1989). These programs are so inconsistent across school systems that it is difficult to evaluate them (Hayes, 1987; Kenney, Guardado, & Brown, 1989; Rosoff, 1989). Excellent curricula are in existence, available for replication. With an improved level of training and quality assurance, these initiatives are fundamental to intelligent health care, whether or not they are seen as "pregnancy prevention." We will describe the effects of a school-linked intervention and some ways in which traditional education can be augmented successfully.

Reproductive Health Interventions

Preventive reproductive health care includes at its core the provision of medical family planning services. Although contraceptive counseling and prescription are key components of this type of intervention, other essential elements include pregnancy testing, sexually transmitted disease testing and treatment (Althaus, 1991; Cates & Rauh, 1985; Hayes, 1987), and the counseling and education related to each of these clinical services. Distribution programs for nonmedical methods are also important (Kirby, Waszak, & Ziegler, 1991); they can increase rates of use and, in the case of condom distribution, are important in efforts to prevent HIV infection and to slow the spread of other sexually transmitted diseases.

There is no doubt that access to contraception brings down pregnancy rates and that a widespread clinic network plays a crucial role in averting large numbers of births and abortions (Forrest, Hermalin, & Henshaw, 1981). The data are clear that the existence of these facilities has been associated with pregnancy prevention and that, in areas that do not have a range of appropriate sites available, fewer adolescents at risk are served. In addition to contraceptive services, pregnancy detection and pregnancy counseling are vital if prenatal care is to be initiated promptly and also to permit a true choice of optimal pregnancy outcome. Finally, the availability of safe and early abortion services is essential to avoid large numbers of unintended births. Following each of these outcomes and following negative pregnancy tests, contraceptive counseling is again an essential reproductive health service.

For adolescents, however, traditional contraceptive facilities have often offered too little, too late. With the risk of pregnancy high in the early months of sexual activity (Zabin et al., 1979) and the tendency of teens not to seek medical care before a crisis occurs (Zabin & Clark, 1981), this population needs more than the categoric clinical services that have often served older women successfully. Clinic services tailored to the needs of teens can have more impact on their behavior than traditional services (Winter & Breckenmaker, 1991). Medical interventions must be combined with intensive outreach and counseling if they are to reach young people in time. General medical care enhanced by explicit counseling about sexuality and contraception can delay sexual onset, reduce frequency of coitus, and improve contraceptive use (Berger et al., 1987; Zabin, Hirsch, Smith, Streett, & Hardy, 1986a).

Some reproductive health interventions have been unable to document an impact on these variables (Herceg-Baron, Furstenberg, Shea, & Mullan, 1986), perhaps because they reach their patients too late. School-based clinics, for example, are designed specifically to reach adolescents early but often fail to do so, especially when their ostensible reproductive health care function is submerged under a broad mandate to deliver comprehensive medical service, when explicit attention to sexual matters is discouraged, or when such discussion and/or the provision of contraceptives is actually prohibited (Dryfoos, 1988; Kirby, Waszak, & Ziegler, 1991).

Even when an increase in contraceptive use is reported, a concomitant decline in the pregnancy rate in the same school population has rarely been documented (Kirby, Waszak, & Ziegler, 1991). The successful program that we will describe here in detail was built on the assumption that medical, educational, counseling, and guidance components are all required and that the goals of postponing sexual onset, decreasing frequency of intercourse, improving contraceptive usage, and preventing pregnancy are not only compatible but mutually reinforcing.

Life Options Interventions

More recent innovations have included attempts to intervene with high-risk populations in ways that increase their life options by improving their self-concept and raising their aspirations and/or by improving their skills, hence the opportunities that will become available to them. The models included in this amorphous group include job training, augmented education and tutoring, mentorship and role-modeling, as well as a range of programs directed specifically at enhancing self-esteem and self-efficacy (Hayes, 1987). Most of the evaluated programs of this type have been targeted at teenage mothers and therefore cannot document the efficacy of such approaches in delaying sexual onset or in preventing a first unintended conception.

Project Redirection, conducted in four cities, demonstrated a significant improvement in school attendance and avoidance of pregnancy among enrollees at 12 months, while the young mothers were still enrolled in the program. At 24 months, after they left the program, the difference was no longer significant between them and a control population in these outcomes (Polit & Kahn, 1985). At 5 years, although fertility was no longer lower among former participants, participation was associated with improved employment, greater self-sufficiency, and, for their children, more favorable cognitive, social, and emotional development (Polit, 1989).

Programs of this kind address well-recognized problems that are not necessarily concerned with "sex" and therefore are not a political challenge. The inherent worth of their objectives makes them easy to support, whether or not they demonstrate an impact on the pregnancy rates that they were often designed to address. Moreover any impact in a high-risk population, even a short one, is not a trivial accomplishment, given how serious the challenge. Such programs must be considered in the light of the odds against which they work; for many reasons, they require further exploration and evaluation before their impact can be judged.

More important, however, is the need to try these programs *before* a first pregnancy or *before* a high-risk behavior is adopted. It is unfortunate that, in some of our most deprived communities, having a first child is the ticket of admission to special initiatives that are closed to those who avoid conception. Therefore a staggering challenge to these interventions is the size of their true target population: To be really "preventive," they would have to reach all young Americans who do not have an optimal environment during their developmental years—and probably many who do. Thus, in the real world, there may be a trade-off between limited preventive strategies addressed to all youth and optimal, high-risk strategies addressed to those who need them most.

PROGRAM EVALUATION

We have suggested that many initiatives have not been subjected to the kind of evaluation they require. Without rigorous assessment, many unsuccessful programs may be duplicated, and the value of many excellent experiments may remain unrecognized. Evaluation, however, is not without cost. In addition to the use of scarce financial resources, researchers face other difficulties when evaluating programs to prevent adolescent pregnancy (for fuller treatment of these issues, see Zabin & Hirsch, 1988). This is not to imply that all creative programs need to be evaluated; it is only to suggest that in the climate of controversy that surrounds these initiatives, it is well to be sure that the human and financial investments are justified.

A program must specify measurable objectives if it is to be successfully evaluated. Not all programs are able (or willing) to make such a commitment. Only if a program is explicitly intended to decrease rates of pregnancy or to delay sexual onset is it appropriate to evaluate it against these criteria. Furthermore, there should be some reason to believe that the program components have a chance of achieving that purpose. It is often the case that programs designed to increase knowledge, or primarily concerned with delivering general health care, are criticized for their lack of success in reducing the pregnancy rate. To expect a clinic in which reproductive health care is only tangential to impact reproductive outcomes is unreasonable. Objectives must be defined, measurable, and feasible in terms of program design if they are to be worth the costs of assessment. In addition to measurable and attainable goals, program managers and staff must be willing to permit the data collection that makes evaluation possible. A specific experimental group, and generally a suitable control population, must be defined. And the initiatives themselves must be carefully articulated.

How, then, can we define an *adolescent pregnancy prevention program?* If sex education programs can vary in content, staff training, duration, materials, and more, so can school-based clinics or life options programs be radically different in conception and design. For example, school clinics may or may not provide contraception, involve outreach, use various methods of education, combine counseling with care, be accessible, have adequate levels of staffing, and be staffed by professionals who have trained with and are committed to adolescents. Each of these variables can be crucial to success or failure, yet only rarely are they the focus of evaluation. The more comprehensive the program, the more difficult it may be to tease out the value of its individual components. It is dangerous to dismiss a promising model because of the failure of any one program—and equally risky to replicate a model without duplicating its most effective innovations.

Given these difficulties, what is to be deduced from the many negative evaluations found in the literature? When an adolescent population is taken as a whole, an evaluation may miss important impacts that only occur within specific subgroups. As mentioned above, the effect of exposure to a program may differ with age, prior sexual experience, ethnicity, gender, and prior exposure to other programs (Eisen et al., 1990). This supports the conclusion that "intervention programs need to be client-specific: one program model does not work equally well for everyone" (p. 269). Sometimes the outcomes that are studied may be too limited and miss important effects. For example, the incidence of first intercourse is not the only measure of increased or decreased sexual activity. Howard and McCabe (1990) found that their outreach program had its major impact on those who had *not* experienced intercourse at the time of exposure to the intervention. Nevertheless there was also an impact on frequency of sexual intercourse, an impact that has equally important implications for health and pregnancy risks. Similarly, Zabin et al. (unpublished) found that their program, which had not hypothesized an impact on the level of sexual activity once coitus was inaugurated, measurably reduced the frequency of coitus among sexually active females.

Counseling interventions are particularly dependent on the personal qualities and skills of counselors. For example, one study comparing contingency-planning counseling with traditional counseling (Namerow, Weatherby, & Williams-Kaye, 1989) found that, although overall there was no impact on contraceptive use and only a short-term impact on pregnancy rates, there were important differences, based on client outcomes, in the efficacy of different counselors. When the least effective contingency-planning counselors were *not* included in the analysis, the differences between the experimental and control groups became more pronounced. When an intervention depends largely on personal interactions, the impact of individual personnel can be critical to evaluation.

A program that shows no significant difference in sexual behavior when the study group is compared to a control group exposed to another program with similar intent but different methods may demonstrate an important impact when the study group is compared to a control group without any exposure at all. Thus there is a difference between those evaluations that try to elucidate the most effective methods of intervention and those that explore the use of any intervention at all.

Negative evaluations can also be very useful tools to revise and improve functioning programs. Kirby, Waszak, and Ziegler (1991) pointed out in their mixed evaluation of school-based clinics that lack of significant change may help identify deficiencies in program services which can readily be changed. Their recommendations, for example, urged explicit priority to pregnancy prevention, more outreach, an attempt to delay and reduce the frequency of sexual activity, identification and targeting of groups in need of specific services, contraceptive availability, effective follow-up, and an emphasis on male responsibility and the efficacy of condoms. These recommendations are not new, but all represent failures in many of the models those authors examined. It would be unfortunate if promising new directions were ignored because of local failures in their implementation; instead, wherever possible—and component by component—successful aspects of new programs might well be replicated.

On the other hand, many well-tested individual program components do not need extensive evaluation; we already know they can complement the services provided by clinics, private clinicians, youth programs, educators, and countless other providers. What they do need is recognition among a broad spectrum of professionals and intelligent integration into the protocols they use with young clients, students, or patients every day.

AN INTERVENTION THAT WORKED:
THE BALTIMORE PROJECT

Between 1981 and 1984, a service and research team designed and implemented a pregnancy prevention program in cooperation with a local junior and senior high school (Zabin, Hardy, Streett, & King, 1984; Zabin et al., 1986a). The program grew from the experience of a group of service providers headed by Janet Hardy, M.D., a pediatrician at the Johns Hopkins School of Medicine, who had been successful in caring for adolescent mothers and their babies and in preventing repeat pregnancies among them. It also grew from research findings at the Johns Hopkins School of Public Health that suggested the importance of intervention before sexual onset or promptly thereafter (Zabin et al., 1979) and the need for free, proximate, and confidential services (Zabin & Clark, 1981). The explicit objectives of the model were to reduce unintended conception through an increase in effective contraceptive use among those who were sexually experienced and to postpone sexual initiation among those who were not.

To reach young people early in their sexual careers, before they became sexually active, it was necessary to reach them in their junior high school (or middle school) years. Waiting until senior high in a population with an early average age of onset will inevitably miss many first pregnancies and preclude the possibility of delaying sexual onset for a high proportion of the group.

The Baltimore program had two components. The first component placed a team—a social worker and occasionally a nurse-midwife or pediatric nurse-practitioner—in the schools, where they were available for class lectures, individual consultation, and small group discussions. The second component was a storefront clinic operated by the hospital, across the street from one school and a few blocks from the other. The staff, known by the students at the school, were available in the clinic in the afternoon. They provided the link to further educational and counseling services and to clinical reproductive health care. Medical services, offered only in the clinic, included pregnancy testing, diagnosis of STDs, contraception, and referrals for other medical complaints. Any student, male or female, was welcome at the school health suite or the "Self Center" (the name the students gave the clinic) at any time, either by appointment or as a walk-in.

Outreach occurred through classroom presentations in the schools. These were important for reaching the largest number of students, some of whom would have only this exposure to the program. The first presentation to each class was used to introduce the program and the staff and to show a film about adolescent pregnancy that raised awareness and was the catalyst for discussion. By the end of the first session, the students knew that they could talk about a range of subjects they had never discussed before with an adult: maturation, sexuality, or other personal concerns. Both in the school and clinic, their response was often immediate.

The most popular aspect of the program was the opportunity for small group discussions, which occurred either on a planned or a spontaneous basis at both sites, including in the clinic waiting area. Staff would use innovative techniques such as educational board games about sexuality and audiovisual materials operated by the students themselves to initiate discussions. They would also bring together groups who shared specific problems, such as late pubertal development or difficult family and peer relationships, or allow informal groups to coalesce around their own issues.

Counseling was available to groups and individuals, and some needy individuals required literally hundreds of contacts for effective assistance (Zabin, Hirsch, Streett, et al., 1988; Zabin & Streett, 1991). An important focus of counseling was to assist teenagers to formulate goals for themselves and explore the ways in which their current behavior would impact on those objectives. The focus on self-discovery and self-direction in no way implied an approach without clear values. Emphasis was placed on delaying sexual activity until older ages, on decreasing the frequency of coitus or the numbers of partners, and on using appropriate methods to prevent pregnancy and sexually transmitted disease. The information and education required to implement these values were woven into every aspect of the program, from classroom presentations, to audiovisual aids, to one-on-one discussions and medical and social work visits.

The program was in effect for a brief 28 months, and yet it demonstrated a dramatic impact on the sexual and contraceptive behavior of the school populations (Zabin, Hirsch, Smith, Streett, & Hardy, 1986b). The services and facilities offered by the program were very popular: Approximately 85% of the students from the schools (or *all* students if allowance is made for chronic absentees) had at least some contact with the program. More than 60% (or three quarters of those attending school) sought out these contacts themselves. By the end of the experimental period, there were dramatic increases in clinic attendance among both males and females, especially among the younger students who most needed improvement. The use of contraception at first and last intercourse improved to a level comparable to or better than that of adult Americans. In every grade in the program schools, including the seventh and eighth grades, fewer than 20% of sexually active female students were unprotected by any method at their most recent coitus. In contrast, at the nonprogram schools only one grade reached such levels of protection; in the other grades, 44% to 49% of the female students at risk were using no method of birth control at all. Use of the pill, a method requiring forethought and clinic attendance, increased at all ages but particularly among the younger groups (Zabin et al., 1986b).

The initiation of sexual activity among those who had not experienced coitus before the program was instituted was delayed from 15 years and 7 months to 16 years and 2 months over the 28-month period. The impact of those 7 months on developmental levels and pregnancy risk is an important one; with so brief an intervention, there was not the time with any one student to effect a greater change. The fact that *any* trend in this direction was demonstrated, however, refutes the charge that such programs encourage early sexual initiation. Clearly they need not.

As a result of these behavior changes, the pregnancy rate among 9th-12th graders in the program schools came down by 30% among those who were exposed to the full length of the program. In the comparison school, the rate rose by 58% during the same time period (Zabin et al., 1986b).

Keys to the success of this program lay in the communication abilities of the staff, the sense of accessibility and possession developed among the students, the dual locus in school and clinic and the bridge the staff created between them, the flexible points of entry into the program, its responsiveness to individual needs, and a philosophy that considered the whole person and the whole school as appropriate foci of intervention (Zabin et al., 1991).

POINTS OF INTERVENTION

If the points of possible intervention are many, so are the required services. Following are some of the most important types of contacts that are needed—some by virtually all adolescents in the United States, others by subgroups at immediate and critical need.

Forestalling Coital Contact

Although programs are needed to delay first intercourse and support abstinence whenever possible, the interventions required to do so are as intensive and specialized as those required to prevent conception. "Just say no" is not an effective exhortation to youngsters caught up in a social milieu in which early sexual initiation is the norm. Acknowledging the early ages at which teenagers mature and become sexually active, providers must respond realistically to the multiple influences on them. This means that frank discussions of sexuality are essential at young ages. However one may wish that the home be the locus for sexuality education, it is apparently necessary that schools take some responsibility for it because the family has often proven an ineffective venue for these discussions (see Chapter 3). A carefully designed site for reproductive health care, a broad mandate to reach young people early, and outreach components to operationalize that mandate are needed if youth are to be helped in time—before they face the decision to initiate or abstain from intercourse. That means their questions and their needs must be addressed as they approach puberty, during their early pubertal years, and frequently thereafter.

Providers who traditionally serve the young, whether as private clinicians or as clinic staff, need to be aware of the sexual issues of concern to this group; they may require specialized training to help them address these concerns before they become problems. The age at which such efforts are required varies, but this should not deter providers from identifying the norms of the populations and the individuals they serve. The more explicit the invitation to the adolescent to open issues of growth, change, and sexuality, the more likely is the young patient to confide. If, on the other hand, those who come in contact with youth await a teenager's own initiative to address these issues, it will probably be too late to affect the timing of sexual onset.

Contraception

Contraceptive prescription is essential for those who are sexually active or expect to be in the near future. Opponents of the provision of contraception, particularly its provision in the school context, often assert that the availability of contraception will encourage promiscuity. There is no evidence that contraception is a prerequisite for sexual activity or that access to it encourages earlier or more frequent coital behavior. In fact, the opposite is true. There is a median delay of 1 year between onset and first contraceptive clinic attendance (Zabin & Clark, 1981). That would hardly suggest that the availability of contraception played a role in sexual initiation. Seeking and using contraception require responsible behavior. Birth control and responsible behavior are not contradictory but complementary; often the best contraceptors have the most control over their sexual lives. Contraception, especially when combined with education and counseling, is central to effective preventive care for adolescents.

Choosing a contraceptive method is not necessarily easy for the teenager or the provider. Making a good choice depends on a provider who is able to evaluate the teenager's life-style, sexual behavior, and maturity and to make effective recommendations while allowing the teenager ultimately to control the decision. At times, the effort to respect the client's autonomy seems contrary to the effort to ensure effective and continued use of the chosen method. For example, it has been found that better continuation rates are associated with more authoritative guidance from the provider, particularly among younger teenagers (Nathanson & Marshall, 1985). Because consistent use is the most important determinant of contraceptive effectiveness, the best choice may not be the method with highest theoretical effectiveness. A good method used regularly is better than an excellent method used sporadically or improperly. Finally, proper use of many methods requires considerable information and sometimes practice. Adolescents use methods even less effectively than older women; their failure and discontinuation rates are high. For all these reasons, thorough counseling must accompany the provision of service if it is to succeed with this group.

Pregnancy Detection and Counseling

Easy access to pregnancy testing services serves three important functions. First, it provides a real choice if a teenager faces an unwanted pregnancy; the later the pregnancy is detected, the more difficult, risky, and expensive is the choice to terminate. In the face of characteristically irregular cycles, fear, denial, and ignorance of sources of care, many teenagers confirm a pregnancy much later than older women and have fewer options and less time to decide as a result. Second, for those deciding to carry to term, early prenatal care is essential to enhance the chances of a well-managed pregnancy and healthy outcome. The earlier a pregnancy is confirmed, the earlier medical care can be encouraged and the health status of the adolescent determined and managed.

Third, pregnancy detection services are an excellent way to identify individuals who are at high risk of conception in the near future. Recent data have shown that teenagers who present at a clinic for a pregnancy test and are *not* pregnant are at extremely high risk of conceiving. In one study, 58% conceived within 18 months of the test; among girls who tested positive and bore a child, 47% conceived in 18 months after delivery; and among those who terminated their pregnancies, 37% conceived in a like period following the procedure (Zabin et al., 1989). Contrary to the assumptions of most providers, the negative test group did not necessarily want to avoid pregnancy, were not especially open to contraceptive counseling because of their "scare," nor likely to become effective contraceptors. This group requires in-depth intervention to explore their reasons for seeking a test, their attitudes toward pregnancy, and their willingness or desire to avoid future conceptions.

Identifying groups at high risk of pregnancy in time to prevent a first conception has been a major stumbling block to the provision of preventive services. It is now clear that this high-risk group is actually presenting at the clinic and can be reached there while they are awaiting the results of their tests. It may even be that the visit is a cry for help; the large percentages of girls in many clinic sites whose tests are negative suggest that this may be the case. Our research describes considerable ambivalence among them toward pregnancy and childbearing. If they are allowed to leave with little or no counseling, they may well reappear in the very near future to experience a positive test.

Abortion

Low-cost, subsidized abortion services are essential if adolescents with unintended conceptions are to have a realistic choice about whether to bear a child. Only about 4% of the adolescent childbearers in a sample presenting for pregnancy tests wanted to conceive; many, before the pregnancy was confirmed, thought that childbearing, not abortion, would be problematic (Zabin et al., 1989). And yet they bore children. Access to abortion among the young and poor is limited by the ability to pay and often by delays in locating necessary funds. Such delays necessitate later abortions, increasing the risks unnecessarily. Although the medical risks of abortion at any stage of gestation are only a fraction of those associated with childbearing, those delays are excessive. Restrictions on access lead many teenagers to bear unintended and often unwanted children who suffer many of the adverse sequelae discussed in Chapter 5. And their mothers have less, not more, chance of forming the nuclear families in the future that are the optimal setting for parents and children alike.

After the procedure, the adolescent needs considerable guidance to help her adopt more protective behavior. For some, the conception was truly a contraceptive failure, but in many cases it was careless use—or nonuse— that led to the pregnancy. Girls who resort to abortion have a much better chance of adopting effective contraception and of avoiding another conception in the 18 months following their outcome than either those with negative tests or those who bear children (Zabin et al., 1989). But the opportunity to help them with intensive contraceptive counseling should not be missed; there may not be another opportunity until it is too late.

Pregnant teenagers require equal nurturing and care whether they choose to carry a pregnancy to term or to terminate it. Too often, teenagers who choose abortion receive less compassion, counseling, and support than those who choose to continue a pregnancy. Both groups are trying to make the best choice for themselves and their families and deserve consistent, in-depth, sensitive counseling. Individual practitioners can be most effective if they evaluate their own skills and prejudices in this area, enhance their counseling skills, enlist the support of team members when possible, and refer clients to other sources of care when necessary.

High-Quality, Obstetrical Care

As suggested in Chapter 5, where this subject is dealt with in some detail, adolescent women are at high risk for poor birth outcomes, but with intensive intervention and comprehensive care, they and their babies stand as good a chance as older women of healthy outcomes. Medical, educational, and social intervention, early and frequent prenatal care, and "high-risk" obstetrical protection at delivery can help avert the difficulties for which adolescent mothers are at risk. Although many of the problems that adolescent girls experience in pregnancy are social rather than biological in origin, they require management just the same. This care is best delivered with a team approach; a medical and nursing staff alone has neither the time nor the expertise to meet all the needs of these patients.

Sexually Transmitted Diseases: Diagnosis and Treatment

The need for discussion of sexually transmitted diseases (STDs), how to detect them and how to avoid them, is becoming increasingly urgent as they reach epidemic proportions. The spread of the HIV virus into the teenage population is probably more common than is recognized; the frequency with which AIDS is diagnosed among men and women in their early 20s suggests how early the virus itself must have been acquired. The need for this care at young ages is clear. Ignorance, unfortunately, is no protection for adolescents, especially in areas where early sexual onset, STDs, and IV drug use are prevalent.

Traditionally, medical practitioners in family planning clinics have confined themselves to history taking, physical examination, and a discussion of side effects or contraindications of birth control. Sexually transmitted diseases and the potential ill effects of early intercourse or multiple partners have often been omitted from medical counseling sessions. (Similarly it is surprising how many STD clinics fail to mention contraception to their obviously sexually active clientele.) Most physicians do not feel that their training equips them to deal with issues of feelings and relationships; for some, discussing the negative risks of sexual activity has been thought to imply a paternalistic or judgmental attitude, to give negative connotations to sexuality, or to impute guilt (Elkins, McNeeley, & Tabb, 1986). The family planning community has also shied away from such discussions in their effort to provide a nonjudgmental and supportive environment. Nevertheless there is a growing realization that the risks of sexually transmitted diseases are so real and the effects so disastrous that such counseling may become an ethical obligation rather than ethically suspect (Elkins et al., 1986; Silber, 1985).

Whether or not clinicians engage in such discourse, however, it is absolutely necessary that those who deal with young people determine whether or not those youngsters are involved in coital activity. If they are, examination for symptoms of disease is essential. The need for prompt treatment to avoid future infection, disease, and infertility makes diagnosis critical, especially in view of the high rates reported in some populations. The fact that many infections are symptom free or have symptoms the adolescent may not recognize puts the responsibility for detection onto the clinician. It also places the responsibility for education in the hands of the family, the school, and the media, a responsibility all of these institutions frequently decline.

Education and Counseling

Programs serving adolescents do best when they integrate medical care into a network of education and counseling. Education about sexuality, health, and parenting, and counseling about values, decision making, pregnancy, and life options can help adolescents avoid many risks—not only those associated with their sexual lives. Education is often offered alone; sometimes counseling and education are offered together. All too often, however, the health care component is missing. If a bridge is provided to preventive and curative medical care, the adolescent can be helped to translate education into preventive behavior. Similarly, medical facilities serving young people do best when they incorporate educational and guidance programs on site; this age group may not recognize their need for these components sufficiently to seek them out once their immediate medical needs are addressed. If not available on site, these services may not be accessed at all.

Topics for discussion, in addition to contraceptive counseling, include the importance of early pregnancy detection to protect adolescents' choices as well as their health, and information on the symptoms of pregnancy so that denial and ignorance are less likely to lead to delay. At a later stage, education and counseling about health and parenting is needed to overcome the high risk that young mothers face of conceiving again in the near future and to protect vulnerable offspring from the potential effects of immature parenting. Teenage parents are in need of support in their parenting efforts; they need role models from whom to learn parenting skills that they may not have acquired through their own early experiences. Thus there is a role for these services at every stage from before sexual onset through contraception, abortion, prenatal and postnatal care, parenting, and once again, prevention.

Services for Young Men

Too few programs address the needs of young men, who are often isolated and excluded from important decisions that affect their own lives and emotional health. If they can be reached early, before 9th or 10th grade, they are often eager and willing to discuss issues of growth, development, and sexuality, to ask questions, and to seek reassurance and guidance (Zabin et al., 1989). Too often, programs designed to serve young women are felt by young men to be inhospitable or uninterested. Intensive outreach is required to attract this group and to test models for assessing and meeting their needs; in the long run, those efforts will help them, their partners, and perhaps their children. There is good evidence that young men maintain longer relationships with their partners at conception than is often believed. Their relationships are not necessarily casual before or after conception. Efforts to reach boys and girls as partners, to help them adopt protective behaviors together, could help them both—whether or not they bear a child.

APPROACHES TO SERVICE PROVISION

Coordination and Continuity

In light of the broad range of services needed by adolescents, these services can have greatest impact if they are coordinated and individualized. Case management and coordination do not necessarily imply a multipurpose setting. Different needs can be met effectively in different places, as long as the settings are equally accessible, both emotionally and physically, to the teenagers in question. Separate settings, such as school and hospital, can be linked through staff members. This idea of "linkage" is a very feasible and cost-effective way of bringing together the broad range of services that adolescents need.

In other settings, familiar providers can supply the continuity that adolescents require if they take the opportunity to build relationships with young people over a period of time so that open communication about sexual concerns can take place at the appropriate developmental period (Zabin, 1990). Family doctors and pediatricians can establish a primary and early relationship with the child, not just his or her parents, and set a pattern legitimating questions about growth, development, and sexual feelings. Consultation in the teenage years can then be part of a continuing, safe, and confidential relationship. In clinics, interventions may be more effective if they build on a strong relationship with one provider. A few situations call for immediate crisis intervention by someone with highly specific training (for example, gynecological examinations for pregnancy or abuse), but many problems—pregnancy options, the results of a pregnancy test, and the repeated contraction of STDS, for example—can be discussed by many different professionals. It may be more helpful to build on an adolescent's trust of one staff member, whenever possible, than to jeopardize that adolescent's willingness to return by trying to transfer this trust to a new and different staff member (Zabin & Streett, 1991).

Because teenagers are not used to discussing personal issues with adults, they are unlikely to raise issues of sexuality directly and often only do so at moments of crisis. If a climate of openness and support exists, providers can indicate their willingness to discuss sensitive matters and not wait for the adolescent to provide the opening. It is a safe assumption that *all* young people have questions and concerns about puberty and sexuality. They are *all* at risk if such concerns are ignored, and they *all* need an opportunity to discuss their questions confidentially. In our experience, when providers indicate their willingness to discuss these issues, young people respond. But if a young person seeks help, however tentatively, and feels rejected or invalidated, he or she may not persist; after a rejection, the adolescent may hesitate to turn to any adult again. The lost opportunity may be the last.

Comprehensive Care

Comprehensive has a number of meanings in adolescent health care. It is used to describe the range of services provided, but these may be a broad range of services meeting a particular need, such as reproductive health care, or a narrow range of services meeting a broad array of needs, such as general health care. For example, routine physicals, medical care for common problems, and health education may be offered in a "comprehensive" clinic that does not address any mental health, counseling, or reproductive health needs. In some cases, when clinics have been given a broad mandate, controversial and sensitive components have been excluded in deference to the demand for more routine services. In this way, many school-based clinics have had no impact on adolescent conception or childbearing because they do not give access to contraception, even though they claim to provide "comprehensive care."

On the other hand, health education, supportive counseling, medical care and referral services, life skills and decision-making training may be offered in a "comprehensive" reproductive health clinic. Such a model assumes that sexual and reproductive health care requires specific attention and expertise but that such needs can only be met with a broad range of services addressing all aspects of the person. In that case, although the focus is categoric, the staff is comprehensive in its training and its orientation.

Thus the notion of "comprehensive" health care can be used in ways that either support or undermine effective reproductive care for teenagers. These interventions may be lost in the effort to provide "comprehensive" health care or may be strengthened by the effort to address a range of adolescent needs, either in a general health clinic or one that focuses on sexuality and reproduction.

It seems clear that the more inclusive the range of services offered to disadvantaged youth, the more successful the program may be in changing attitudes and behavior. Indeed comprehensive service may be an excellent environment for the provision of reproductive health care and counseling to all adolescents, if these services are explicitly included. A range of nonreproductive services may also provide the diversification that helps maintain anonymity for teenagers seeking advice about sexual matters.

That does not mean that every service need necessarily be offered in the same setting. Each setting (school, clinic, hospital, or office) may be suited to providing some but not all services and may be linked with other settings to complete the circle. Complementary interventions can be available in each place, if the linkage is real. Whatever the social or economic group of adolescents served, however, the notion of providing "health" service *without* contraceptive service is a poor one. Not only are many patients lost when referrals are required but the message itself also is destructive. There is too much fear of contraception and ambivalence about its use among women of all ages in the United States. A respected health center that does not make contraceptive methods available compounds the negative attitudes that are the primary barrier to effective contraceptive use among American women today. That negative message is not consistent with the responsible behavior we are trying to instill among sexually active adolescents.

Confidentiality

Reassurance of confidential consultation, without legal interference in the right of the provider to ensure privacy, is essential to effective intervention. It has been shown in many studies that adolescents require a guarantee of confidentiality before they are comfortable seeking care. At every stage of sexual experience, from concerns about physical development to decisions about pregnancy, adolescents want their confidence protected and often voice the fear that their parents or family members will "find out."

This does not suggest that most young people do not turn to their parent(s) for help. They do. In one study, we have shown that over 91% of young black women at 17 years of age or below who presented for pregnancy tests had already told their mothers (or surrogate mothers if raised by someone else) that they suspected a pregnancy *before* presenting for the test (Zabin, Hirsch, Raymond, & Emerson, 1992). Before the outcome decision was made, the percentage rose still higher. In fact, even among the girls who did not live with their mothers, 65% had sought out their mothers to tell them. Thus the vast majority of adolescents want to confide in parents and will do so if that is a reasonable option. If they do not, there is probably a rational reason for their reticence. In most situations, providers will encourage an adolescent to communicate with his or her parents; in fact, it is often through the work of such a counselor that communication is opened. But the final decision must be left to teenagers themselves if they are not to be pushed away from the very services that can help them most.

Confidentiality is not only a policy decided at the level of legislation and institutional management but also is an attitude that can be conveyed at each encounter with a provider. In close-knit communities or where an office or clinic has provided care to whole families for a long time, the teenager may feel vulnerable when seeking services about sensitive matters. On the other hand, specialty clinics, such as family planning or prenatal clinics, pose a different challenge, because teenagers may feel that the purpose of their visit is all too obvious. Once again, the role of a comprehensive facility is underscored, as long as the staff in such a site can establish a sense of privacy and personal respect.

Identifying High-Risk Individuals

If behaviors that plague young people at risk are found to cluster not only in certain individuals but also in certain settings, that is a good argument for seeking to substitute alternative *patterns* of behavior rather than treating each dangerous activity as a separate problem. Behaviors are adopted because they fulfill needs, because—however destructive—they serve some positive purpose in the young person's life (Jessor, 1992). Therefore it is not enough to tell them that the behavior puts them at risk or puts others at risk; they may be well aware of that. It may be much more useful to make available ways to meet those needs with other, more beneficial, activities. Clearly, in many communities, that will require basic structural change. All a program can do is offer some limited but useful alternatives.

The evidence that substance use and early sexual onset are statistically associated within gender/race subgroups (Zabin, Hardy, et al., 1986) suggests that facilities addressing one of these areas might well incorporate others. Because both are symptoms of need rather than separate "problems," early intervention with supportive educational and emotional treatment is indicated. Once in adolescence, each manifestation of risk requires trained, professional guidance; the family planning counselor and the drug counselor have skills of their own. But diagnosis and contact can be made at the same site. It is hoped that whichever route is taken to help the young person acquire self-respect and control over his or her life will, in the process, affect other behaviors as well.

Individuals at highest risk are most likely to be lost to any intervention at an early age because of early school termination and the likelihood that their subsequent life-style will distance them from previously established sources of care. This is true particularly for young men who are likely to compound their risks after leaving school and who rarely encounter service institutions with the possible exception of STD clinics. It is therefore essential to develop systems for identifying high-risk individuals, preferably in the early school years. We have shown that late elementary or early junior high school years are appropriate times for discussions of pubertal development and sexual responsibility; at early ages, young men are most open to these areas of intervention. Once identified early, they must be provided with intensive support and guidance before unacceptable behaviors are adopted and before they leave the school setting in large numbers. Although massive and early intervention sounds like an expensive option, it is justified both in human and economic terms; all that we know about the clustering of high-risk behaviors suggests that in time these youth will command resources for correction and punishment that would have been more productively spent for prevention.

Proximate, Free, and Flexible Care

Teenagers do not have the funds to pay for services or the confidence or wherewithal to seek transportation to distant or unfamiliar sites. Services must be available close to where teenagers spend their time; schools, shopping centers, and storefronts all offer good locations for special facilities. Sources of care that served the teenager through childhood, if they can give assurance of confidentiality, are very important, as they are familiar and accessible; they can provide continuity of care, which has been shown to accelerate utilization (Zabin & Clark, 1981).

Whatever its location, any program that hopes to serve the teenage population must invest in outreach. Teenagers need to know not only where the program is, what is offered, and what it costs (preferably that it is free) but also that it is open to them and offers a caring and confidential environment. If female clinicians are available to young women, that should be made known; many girls say that they choose a clinic for that reason (Zabin & Clark, 1981). If education, counseling, and medical services are provided in different sites, all must be easily accessible, and the referral system must be managed so that clients are not lost between them.

Teenagers are often stymied by limited and inconvenient clinic hours. Owing to their crisis orientation and natural impatience, they are unlikely to seek help if it has once been refused at a time of need. Although appropriate hours are often difficult for programs to arrange, a facility that can accommodate the needs of clients is most likely to be effective. An open-door policy, with walk-ins accepted as quickly as possible, appointments available in the not-too-distant future, some evening and weekend hours, and constructive use of waiting time is most likely to attract teenage clients. In turn, it has been established that geographic areas with a wide range of different but accessible services are the areas in which a higher proportion of at-risk teens are served.

Group Discussion and Counseling

Teenagers spontaneously form groups and are often dependent on peers for security. Although individual counseling is an essential component of reproductive health care, group discussions should probably play a more prominent role than they do. Small groups can be used to explore issues within a close group of confidants or to address the needs of adolescents with specific problems in common. The school setting is well suited to this sort of intervention, but the principle that teenagers can be more at ease in a group than in individual sessions, particularly for discussions of sexuality, is transferable to the office or clinic. Providers of all types may find ways to encourage small group discussions and may find that they are a cost-efficient way to manage the educational and counseling process (Zabin, Hirsch, Smith, et al., 1988). In clinic sites, an educator can offer them informally in the waiting room or—with an eye to patient flow—at appointed times and places in the course of the visit. Even in private practice such sessions can be useful: In offices that include several family practitioners or pediatricians, the doctors may find that a single educator or social worker can relieve them of hours of expensive individual consultation. The youngest groups of adolescents, uneasy about seeking care and counsel alone, may find such options particularly helpful.

Focus on Staff

The essential ingredient of any program is its staff. A well-trained, diverse, and committed staff will make the largest contribution to a program's success. A strong team of professionals with a variety of skills not only can meet an adolescent's various needs but also can provide support to one another in fulfilling roles with which they are less familiar. For many medical clinicians, a social worker, educator, or guidance counselor may be the most appropriate team member and may represent the best use of time, resources, and skills. Many providers are involved in the training of new professionals. Unfortunately the focus of much of that training is on acute care, particularly in medical and nursing specialties; that means these professionals have little experience in preventive intervention. An effort must be made to address issues of preventive care and to develop the necessary skills during the training of house staff and other health care personnel.

The place of values in sexuality education and in family planning counseling has long been the subject of debate. It is hoped that providers who interact with adolescents will try to fit their personal and professional judgment within the framework of value-free guidance. Such an ideal may be unattainable; family planning counselors and educators in the field of sexuality inevitably do their work under some assumptions about its purpose and value—assumptions that include a particular vision of the place of sexuality in social behavior in general and the needs of teenagers in particular (Joffe, 1986; Nathanson, 1991). Different professionals see the role for their own values very differently. Some regard the adolescent as less than competent and hope to be trusted by adolescents "to act in the interest of the selves that they would be if they were mature" (Silber, 1985, p. 92). Others feel obliged to support the client's decisions regardless of their personal judgment. It would be unwise to assume that all service providers are appropriate to the tasks outlined here. Some providers find it difficult to approach options counseling from a neutral standpoint; the degree of skill and training required for this task is usually underestimated. But beyond their level of skill, there remains a larger question of moral and social orientation. To ask a professional who finds early sexual onset "immoral" to be objective and nonjudgmental in his or her counseling may be fruitless. A manager, of course, has the responsibility to evaluate the fit between a staff member and a specific task, but just as important, a service provider has the obligation to decline to serve in a setting with which his or her own philosophy puts that provider at odds. Although a program can be based on a clear value system, it cannot communicate the caring and support young people require unless the staff truly *do* care and unless they are intellectually and emotionally open to the needs and the confidences their clients share.

CONCLUSION

Intervening with adolescents can take place at many points: before sexual onset, for contraception, after conception (through options counseling and services), to parenting, and again, to the delivery of preventive contraceptive services. Successful models for service delivery involve a range of provider specialties; unfortunately the political will to make these services available to those in greatest need has not been demonstrated.

Professionals who serve adolescents are well placed to take on a public role, to speak out for the needs of this population, and to clarify the issues that are often either polarized or ignored. It is regrettable that a small minority of Americans make issues of teenage sexuality seem more controversial than they are. Well-informed providers can be the voice of reason in these debates. They are better equipped than most citizens to explain the etiology of adolescent behavior and to focus attention on the needs of this age group. They can define the appropriate role for individual intervention, on the one hand, and structural change, on the other. And they can testify to the need for a wide range of services if the problems encountered by one generation are not to become the risk factors that plague the next.

7

CONCLUSION

We suggested at the outset that there are two quite different problems of adolescent sexual activity and pregnancy in the United States today. One involves sexual initiation in the midteens and accidental pregnancy that generally terminates in abortion. The other involves sexual onset in the early pubertal or postpubertal years and accidental conception during the teen years, also often resulting in unintended abortion but very frequently in childbearing. Whereas the first problem knows no geographic, social, or economic boundaries, the second has become a familiar pattern in our most disadvantaged communities.

Where the family, the social institutions, and the larger environment are generally protective of the adolescent, and where throughout childhood the young person has developed a strong sense of self and of his or her present and future potential, adolescents generally have the ability to avoid behaviors that put that future at risk. Or if it is placed at risk, they are likely to make decisions that return them to the positive developmental trajectory on which they have embarked. Of course within any social or economic environment, there may well be characteristics of the family or the individual life course that predispose a child to risk, but when the environment is optimal, these problem situations are in some measure aberrational. Thus very early sexual onset is rare in these settings, and where conception does occur in the teen years, it is usually terminated in abortion.

In our poorest neighborhoods, however, there are few resources to protect children from risk either within the family or in the larger environment. Personal characteristics protective against risk have little chance to develop—characteristics such as positive scholastic achievement and aspirations, a strong sense of self and future options, and the ability to relate to successful, proximate role models. The normative peer behaviors that the adolescent does observe within the community have been motivated by the same needs that motivate him or her. Many of the adolescent behaviors that are seen only in negative terms by adults, because they seem to threaten a healthy transition to adulthood, actually serve positive needs that are not otherwise served in the young person's social setting. When that setting fails large numbers of young people so that they collectively adopt similar risk behaviors, we call that setting a high-risk neighborhood, and "risky" activities become not aberrations but normative behavior.

The Need for Intervention

Who, then, is in need of services if adverse effects of early sexual contact, early pregnancy, and early childbearing are to be averted? Both males and females in all social and economic groups and in several age groups require some level of intervention. For all of them, an improved level of sexuality education within the schools is the sine qua non of responsible behavior. There is strong support for these efforts from parents all over the country. It is hoped that, especially in the context of the AIDS and HIV epidemic, the form that education takes will not be so negative and so polemical that it has a negative impact on a vital and positive aspect of human life. Clear, unbiased, and specific information is a first step, without which few interventions can succeed. Coupled with an ability to understand consequences and to make and maintain decisions about personal behavior, it can provide young people with some of the skills they need to protect themselves.

To the extent that parents can be helped to communicate better with their children of all ages, that initiative would certainly be desirable. But even if successful, such a program can in no way relieve the educational system of a central role in imparting information and in developing interpersonal skills from the primary through the high school years. Nor can it relieve health professionals who come in contact with the growing child from their obligation to represent a source of confidential and sensitive care with respect to the developmental and sexual issues that concern all young people as they approach and experience puberty and adolescence.

For those who are sexually active or expect to be in the near future, a source of contraceptive care and the diagnosis and treatment of sexually transmitted disease are basic health service requirements. For the older males and females among them who are about to or have recently initiated coitus, that care, delivered in an appropriate setting with an opportunity for education and counseling, is probably sufficient.

For younger adolescents, for older teens who have a history of coital contact, and for young women who have already experienced a pregnancy, much more is required. For them, the wide range of services discussed in Chapter 6 are all necessary, and all must be delivered in an appropriate way for each age group. If maturity in one area does not predict maturity in another, interventions based on chronological age or even on gynecological age may not be appropriate to young people at the very time they are most in need.

An Interactive Model

The processes of child and adolescent development, subject to influences that interact within and across generations, have complex effects on the sexual behaviors, attitudes, and beliefs of young teenagers. We have suggested that only a model that takes account of the sequential interactions of biological *and* environmental factors can help us appreciate the diverse developmental courses expressed in their sexual lives and the normal pubertal pressures on them to engage in coital behavior. Only such a model can make it clear that the resources required to resist those pressures are very great, whether in terms of inner resources or in terms of the reward structures that make resistance attractive. These resources are not available to large numbers of adolescents in the United States today.

Although young people grow within a context socially defined by family and community and individually defined by characteristics such as health, hormones, and evolving self-concept, they are also bombarded by the mixed messages of a society that has considerable uneasiness with "sex." Caught in this maze, it is little wonder that American teenagers produce rates of sexual activity, sexually transmitted disease, and accidental pregnancy that remain—or have risen—unacceptably high. Nor is it surprising that abortion rates and rates of unintended childbearing among adolescents compare adversely with those of any other developed country.

All these statistics have been in the public eye for some time; the country's failure to act is not predicated on blindness to problems of youth and reproductive health. But the cultural "uneasiness" toward sex has made it possible for politicians with little concern for young people or for their futures to make them pawns in political battles that can only do them harm. Arguments about parental notification, health care funding, and the provision of medical services and counsel have no place on the political agenda; the data on which these professional decisions should be predicated are in the public domain.

Can interventions help? There is good evidence that they can. One hopeful sign is the fact that programs that build trust and offer acceptable, accessible, and appropriate services can make a difference (Hardy & Zabin, 1991; Hayes, 1987; Zabin et al., 1986a). Although childhood is a better time to intervene, adolescence is not too late. The Head Start program showed that the academic effects of birth status and economic setting can be ameliorated by early intervention. But there is good and growing evidence that an improvement in life circumstances at any time during a child's young life can change important aspects of his or her development; Furstenberg and Brooks-Gunn (1987) confirmed the effects of changed maternal status on offspring throughout childhood and adolescence. Even preventing a *second* unintended conception to a teenage mother can help minimize the stresses on several generations: the young mother, her child, and her primary family. The potential for intervention is therefore great.

There is a danger that, by asserting the power of individual programs independently to make measurable differences in young people's lives, one is relieving the larger society of the responsibility for fundamental and structural change. We think not. There is too much to be done. The range of categorical services that adolescents require are suggested above. But beyond those services are the desperate and multiple needs of young people without education or jobs, without resources or hope. Until fundamental changes are brought about, any professional in contact with youth, any educator with programs for youth, any provider with services for youth can find positive ways to intervene. And any citizen, legislator, administrator, or parent can find constructive ways to support that endeavor.

REFERENCES

Alan Guttmacher Institute (AGI). (1991). *Teenage sexual and reproductive behavior* (Facts in Brief). New York: Author.

Althaus, F. A. (1991). An ounce of prevention . . . STDs and women's health. *Family Planning Perspectives, 23,* 173-177.

Apter, D., & Vihko, R. (1977). Serum pregnenolone, progesterone, 17-hydroxyprogesterone, testosterone and 5(alpha)-dihydro testosterone during female puberty. *Journal of Clinical Endocrinology and Metabolism, 45,* 1039-1048.

Bauman, K. E., & Udry, J. R. (1981). Subjective expected utility and adolescent sexual behavior. *Adolescence, 16,* 527-535.

Bell, T. A., & Holmes, K. K. (1984). Age-specific risks of syphilis, gonorrhea, and hospitalized pelvic inflammatory disease in sexually experienced U.S. women. *Sexually Transmitted Diseases, 11,* 291-295.

Bentler, P. M. (1968). Heterosexual behaviors (1 and 2). *Behavioral and Social Research, 6,* 21-30.

Berger, D. K., Perez, G., Kyman, W., Perez, L., Garson, J., Menendez, M., Bistritz, J., Blanchard, H., & Dombrowski, C. (1987). Influence of family planning counseling in an adolescent clinic on sexual activity and contraceptive use. *Journal of Adolescent Health Care, 8,* 436-440.

Bernard, J. (1975). Adolescence and socialization for motherhood: In S. Dragastin & G. Elder (Eds.), *Adolescence in the life cycle: Psychological change and social context* (pp. 227-252). New York: Hemisphere.

Bernstein, A. C., & Cowan, P. A. (1975). Children's concepts of how people get babies. *Child Development, 46,* 77-91.

Billy, J. O. G., Rodgers, J. L., & Udry, J. R. (1984). Adolescent sexual behavior and friendship choice. *Social Forces, 62,* 653-678.

Billy, J. O. G., & Udry, J. R. (1983). *The effects of age and pubertal development on adolescent sexual behavior.* Unpublished manuscript, University of North Carolina, Carolina Population Center, Chapel Hill.

Billy, J. O. G., & Udry, J. R. (1985a). The influence of male and female best friends on adolescent sexual behavior. *Adolescence, 20,* 21-31.

Billy, J. O. G., & Udry, J. R. (1985b). Patterns of adolescent friendship and effects on sexual behavior. *Social Psychology Quarterly, 48,* 27-31.

Bojlen, K., & Bentzon, M. W. (1968). The influence of climate and nutrition on age at menarche: A historical review and a modern hypothesis. *Human Biology, 40,* 69-85.

Boxill, N. A. (1987). How would you feel . . . ? Clinical interviews with black adolescent mothers. In H. Jones (Ed.), *The black adolescent parent* (pp. 41-52). New York: Haworth.

Boyce, W. T., Schaeffer, C., & Uitti, C. (1985). Permanence and change: Psychosocial factors in the outcome of adolescent pregnancy. *Social Science and Medicine, 21,* 1279-1287.

Brady, J. P., & Levitt, E. E. (1965). The scalability of sexual experiences. *Psychological Record, 15,* 275-279.

Brooks-Gunn, J., & Furstenberg, F. F. (1989). Adolescent sexual behavior. *American Psychologist, 44,* 249-257.

Brown, S. S. (1989). Drawing women into prenatal care. *Family Planning Perspectives, 21,* 73-80.

Buck, C., & Stavraky, K. (1967). The relationship between age at menarche and age at marriage among childbearing women. *Human Biology, 39,* 93-102.

Bureau of the Census. (1984). *Marital status and living arrangements* (Current Population Reports. Series P-20, No. 389.) Washington, DC: U.S. Department of Commerce.

Bureau of the Census. (1985). *Statistical abstracts of the United States* (105th ed.). Washington, DC: U.S. Department of Commerce.

Bureau of the Census. (1986). *Statistical abstracts of the United States* (106th ed.). Washington, DC: U.S. Department of Commerce.

Card, J. J., & Wise, L. L. (1978). Teenage mothers and teenage fathers: The impact of early childbearing on parents' personal and professional lives. *Family Planning Perspectives, 10,* 199-205.

Cates, W., Jr. (1980). Adolescent abortions in the United States. *Journal of Adolescent Health Care, 1,* 18-25.

Cates, W., Jr., & Rauh, J. L. (1985). Adolescents and sexually transmitted diseases: An expanding problem. *Journal of Adolescent Health Care, 6,* 257-261.

Cates, W., Jr., Schultz, K. F., & Grimes, D. A. (1983). The risks associated with teenage abortion. *New England Journal of Medicine, 309,* 621-624.

Cherlin, A. J. (1989). The weakening link between marriage and the care of children. *Family Planning Perspectives, 20,* 302-306.

Cutler, W. B., Garcia, C. R., & Krieger, A. M. (1979). Infertility and age at first coitus: A possible relationship. *Journal of Biosocial Science, 11,* 425.

Damon, W., & Hart, D. (1982). The development of self-understanding from infancy through adolescence. *Child Development, 53,* 841-864.

. Danielson, R., Marcy, S., Plunkett, A., Wiest, W., & Greenlick, M. R. (1990). Reproductive health counseling for young men: What does it do? *Family Planning Perspectives, 22,* 115-121.

Dawson, D. A. (1986). The effects of sex education on adolescent behavior. *Family Planning Perspectives, 18,* 162-170.

DiClemente, R. J. (1990). The emergence of adolescents as a risk group for human immunodeficiency virus infection. *Journal of Adolescent Research, 5,* 7-17.

Drillien, C. M. (1964). *The growth and development of the prematurely born infant.* Baltimore: Williams & Wilkins.

Dryfoos, J. G. (1983). Family planning clinics—a story of growth and conflict. *Family Planning Perspectives, 15,* 282-297.

Dryfoos, J. G. (1988). School-based health clinics: Three years of experience. *Family Planning Perspectives, 20,* 193-200.

Edelman, M. W. (1987). *Families in peril: An agenda for social change.* Cambridge, MA: Harvard University Press.

Eisen, M., Zellman, G. L., & McAlister, A. L. (1990). Evaluating the impact of a theory-based sexuality and contraceptive education program. *Family Planning Perspectives, 22,* 261-271.

Elkind, D. (1967). Egocentrism in adolescence. *Child Development, 38,* 1025-1034.

Elkind, D. (1975). Recent research on cognitive development in adolescence. In S. Dragastin & G. Elder (Eds.), *Adolescence in the life cycle: Psychological change and social context* (pp. 49-61). New York: John Wiley.

Elkins, T. E., McNeeley, S. G., & Tabb, T. (1986). A new era in contraceptive counseling for early adolescents. *Journal of Adolescent Health Care, 7,* 405-408.

Eriksen, E. H. (1965). Identity versus identity diffusion. In P. Mussen, J. J. Conger, & J. Kagan (Eds.), *Readings in child development and personality* (pp. 435-441). New York: Harper & Row.

Evans, R. C. (1987). Adolescent sexual activity, pregnancy, and childrearing: Attitudes of significant others as risk factors. In H. Jones (Ed.), *The black adolescent parent* (pp. 75-93). New York: Haworth.

Forrest, J. D. (1986). *Proportion of U.S. women ever pregnant before age 20: A research note.* Unpublished manuscript, Alan Guttmacher Institute (AGI), New York.

Forrest, J. D., Hermalin, A., & Henshaw, S. (1981). The impact of family planning clinic programs on adolescent pregnancy. *Family Planning Perspectives, 13,* 109-116.

Forrest, J. D., & Silverman, J. (1989). What public school teachers teach about preventing pregnancy, AIDS and sexually transmitted diseases. *Family Planning Perspectives, 21,* 65-72.

Forrest, J. D., & Singh, S. (1990). The sexual and reproductive behavior of American women, 1982-1988. *Family Planning Perspectives, 22,* 206-214.

Frank, D. B. (1983). *Deep blue funk and other stories: Portraits of teenage parents.* Chicago: Ounce of Prevention Fund.

Frisch, R. E. (1972). Weight at menarche. Similarity for well-nourished and undernourished girls at differing ages, and evidence for historical consistency. *Pediatrics, 50,* 445-450.

Frisch, R. E., & Revell, R. (1971). Height and weight at menarche and a hypothesis of menarche. *Archives of Disease in Childhood, 46,* 695-701.

Furstenberg, F. F., Jr. (1976). *Unplanned parenthood: The social consequences of teenage childbearing.* New York: Free Press.

Furstenberg, F. F., Jr., Brooks-Gunn, J., & Morgan, S. P. (1987). Adolescent mothers and their children in later life. *Family Planning Perspectives, 19,* 142-151.

Goldman, R. J., & Goldman, J. D. G. (1982). How children perceive the origin of babies and the roles of mothers and fathers in procreation: Cross-national study. *Child Development, 53,* 491-504.

Goldsmith, S., Gabrielson, M. O., Gabrielson, I., & Matthews V. (1972). Teenagers, sex and contraception. *Family Planning Perspectives, 4,* 32-38.

Grimes, D. A., & Cates, W. (1979). Complications from legally induced abortion: A review. *Obstetrics Gynecology Survey, 34,* 177-191.

Hardy, J. B., & Zabin, L. S. (1991). *Adolescent pregnancy in an urban environment: Issues, programs and evaluation.* Washington, DC: The Urban Institute Press.

Hauser, S., Powers, S. I., Noam, G. G., Jacobson, A. M., Weiss, B., & Follansbee, D. J. (1984). Familial contexts of adolescent ego development. *Child Development, 55,* 195-213.

Hayes, C. D. (Ed.). (1987). *Risking the future: Adolescent sexuality, pregnancy and childbearing* (Vol. 1). Washington, DC: National Academy Press.

Herceg-Baron, R., Furstenberg, F. F., Jr., Shea, J., & Harris, K. M. (1986). Supporting teenagers' use of contraceptives: A comparison of clinic services. *Family Planning Perspectives, 18,* 61-66.

Hirsch, M. B., & Zelnik, M. (1985). Contraceptive method switching among American female adolescents, 1979. *Journal of Adolescent Health Care, 6,* 1-7.

Hofferth, S. L. (1987). Factors affecting initiation of sexual intercourse. In S. L. Hofferth & C. D. Hayes (Eds.), *Risking the future: Adolescent sexuality, pregnancy and childbearing* (Vol. 2, pp. 7-35). Washington, DC: National Academy Press.

Hofferth, S. L., & Hayes, C. D. (Eds.). (1987). *Risking the future: Adolescent sexuality, pregnancy and childbearing* (Vol. 2). Washington, DC: National Academy Press.

Hofferth, S. L., Kahn, J. R., & Baldwin, W. (1987). Premarital sexual activity among U.S. teenage women over the past three decades. *Family Planning Perspectives, 19,* 46-53.

Hogan, D. P., & Kitagawa, E. M. (1985). The impact of social status, family structure and neighborhood on the fertility of black adolescents. *American Journal of Sociology, 90,* 825-855.

Horwitz, S. M., Klerman, L. V., Kuo, H. S., & Jekel, J. F. (1991). Intergenerational transmission of school-age parenthood. *Family Planning Perspectives, 23,* 168-177.

Howard, M., & McCabe, J. B. (1990). Helping teenagers postpone sexual involvement. *Family Planning Perspectives, 22,* 21-26.

Institute of Medicine. (1985). *Preventing low birthweight.* Washington, DC: National Academy Press.

Jessor, R. (1992). Risk behavior in adolescence: A psychosocial framework for understanding and action. In D. E. Rogers & E. Ginzberg (Eds.), *Adolescents at risk: Medical and social perspectives* (pp. 19-34). (Cornell University Medical College Seventh Conference on Health Policy). Boulder, CO: Westview.

Jessor, R., & Jessor, S. L. (1977). *Problem behavior and psychosocial development: A longitudinal study of youth.* New York: Academic Press.

Joffe, C. (1986). *The regulation of sexuality: Experiences of family planning workers.* Philadelphia: Temple University Press.

Johnston, F. E. (1974). Control of age at menarche. *Human Biology, 46,* 159-171.

Johnston, F. E., Roche, A. F., Schell, L. M., & Wettenhall, H.N.B. (1975). Critical weight at menarche. *American Journal of Diseases of Children, 129,* 19-23.

Jones, E. F., Forrest, J. D., Goldman, N., & Henshaw, S. K. (1985). Teenage pregnancy in developed countries: Determinants and policy implications. *Family Planning Perspectives, 17,* 53-63.

Jones, E. F., Forrest, J. D., Goldman, N., Henshaw, S., Lincoln, R., Rosoff, J. I., Westoff, C. F., & Wulf, D. (1986). *Teenage pregnancy in industrialized countries.* New Haven, CT: Yale University Press.

Jones, E. F., Forrest, J. D., Henshaw, S. K., Silverman, J., & Torres, A. (1988). Unintended pregnancy, contraceptive practice and family planning services in developed countries. *Family Planning Perspectives, 20,* 53-67.

Katchadourian, H. (1980). Adolescent sexuality. *Pediatric Clinics of North America, 27,* 17-28.

Kellam, S. G., Adams, R. G., Brown, C. H., et al. (1982). The long-term evolution of the family structure of teenage and older mothers. *Journal of Marriage and the Family, 42,* 539-554.

Kellam, S. G., Ensminger, M. E., & Turner, R. J. (1977). Family structure and the mental health of children. *Archives of General Psychiatry, 34,* 1012-1022.

Kenny, A. M., Guardado, S., & Brown, L. (1989). Sex education and AIDS education in the schools: What states and large school districts are doing. *Family Planning Perspectives, 12,* 56-64.

Kinsey, A. C., Pomeroy, W. B., & Martin, C. E. (1948). *Sexual behavior in the human male.* Philadelphia: W. B. Saunders.

Kinsey, A. C., Pomeroy, W. B., Martin, C. E., & Gebhard, P. (1953). *Sexual behavior in the human female.* Philadelphia: W. B. Saunders.

Kirby, D. (1984). *Sexuality education: An evaluation of programs and their effects.* Santa Cruz, CA: Network.

Kirby, D., Barth, R. P., Leland, N., & Fetro, J. V. (1991). Reducing the risk: Impact of a new curriculum on sexual risk-taking. *Family Planning Perspectives, 23,* 253-263.

Kirby, D., Waszak, C., & Ziegler, J. (1991). Six school-based clinics: Their reproductive health services and impact on sexual behavior. *Family Planning Perspectives, 23,* 6-16.

Kohlberg, L. (1964). Development of moral character and moral ideology. In M. L. Hoffman & L. W. Hoffman (Eds.), *Review of child development research* (Vol. 1, pp. 383-431). New York: Russell Sage.

Litt, I. F., & Cohen, M. I. (1973). Age of menarche: A changing pattern and its relationship to ethnic origin and delinquency. *Journal of Pediatrics, 82,* 288-289.

Luker, K. (1975). *Taking chances: Abortion and the decision not to contracept.* Berkeley: University of California Press.

Marshall, W. A., & Tanner, J. M. (1974). Puberty. In J. A. Davis & J. Dobbing (Eds.), *Scientific foundations of pediatrics* (pp. 124-162). Philadelphia: W. B. Saunders.

Marsiglio, W. (1987). Adolescent fathers in the United States: Their initial living arrangements, marital status and educational outcome. *Family Planning Perspectives, 19,* 245-251.

Marsiglio, W., & Mott, F. L. (1986). The impact of sex education on sexual activity, contraceptive use and premarital pregnancy among American teenagers. *Family Planning Perspectives, 18,* 151-162.

McAnarney, E. R. (1987). Young maternal age and adverse neonatal outcome. *American Journal of Disease Control, 141,* 1053-1059.

McLanahan, S. S. (1983). Family structure and stress: A longitudinal comparison of two-parent and female-headed families. *Journal of Marriage and the Family, 43,* 347-357.

McLanahan, S. S. (1985). Family structure and the reproduction of poverty. *American Journal of Sociology, 90,* 873-901.

Modell, J. (1989). *Into one's own: From youth to adulthood in the United States, 1920-1975.* Berkeley: University of California Press.

Modell, J., Furstenberg, F. F., Jr., & Hershberg, T. (1978). Social change and transitions to adulthood in historical perspective. In M. Gordon (Ed.), *The American family in social historical perspective* (2nd ed., pp. 192-219). New York: St. Martin's.

Moore, K. A., Nord, C. W., & Peterson, J. L. (1989). Nonvoluntary sexual activity among adolescents. *Family Planning Perspectives, 21,* 110-114.

Moore, K. A., Wenk, D., Hofferth, S. L., & Hayes, C. D. (1987). Statistical appendix, Table 3-1. In S. L. Hofferth & C. D. Hayes (Eds.), *Risking the future* (Vol 2, pp. 414-415). Washington, DC: National Academy Press.

Morrison, D. M. (1985). Adolescent contraceptive behavior: A review. *Psychological Bulletin, 98,* 538-568.

Mosher, W. D., & McNally, J. W. (1991). Contraceptive use at first premarital intercourse: United States, 1965-1988. *Family Planning Perspectives, 23,* 108-116.

Mott, F. L. (1983). *Fertility-related data in the 1982 National Longitudinal Survey of Work Experience of Youth: An evaluation of data quality and some preliminary analytical results.* Columbus: Ohio State University, Center for Human Resource Research.

Mott, F. L., & Marsiglio, W. (1985). Early childbearing and the completion of high school. *Family Planning Perspectives, 17,* 234-237.

Namerow, P. B., Weatherby, N., & Williams-Kaye, J. (1989). The effectiveness of contingency-planning counseling. *Family Planning Perspectives, 21,* 115-119.

Nathanson, C. (1991). *Dangerous passage: The social control of sexuality in women's adolescence.* Philadelphia: Temple University Press.

Nathanson, C. A., & Marshall, H. B. (1985). The influence of client-provider relationships on teenage women's subsequent use of contraception. *American Journal of Public Health, 75,* 33-38.

National Center for Health Statistics. (1988). *Advance report of final natality statistics, 1986* (Monthly Vital Statistics Report 37[3]). Hyattsville, MD: U.S. Department of Health and Human Services.

Newcomer, S. F., & Udry, J. R. (1984). Mothers' influence on the sexual behavior of teenage children. *Journal of Marriage and the Family, 46,* 477-485.

Newcomer, S. F., & Udry, J. R. (1985). Parent-child communication and adolescent sexual behavior. *Family Planning Perspectives, 17,* 169-174.

Nicolson, A. B., & Hanley, C. (1953). Indices of physiological maturity: Deviation and interrelationships. *Child Development, 24,* 3-38.

Piaget, J. (1972). Intellectual evolution from adolescence to adulthood. *Human Development, 15,* 1-12.

Pierke, K., Kockett, G., & Dittmar, F. (1974). Psychosexual stimulation and plasma testosterone in man. *Archives of Sexual Behavior, 3,* 577-584.

Polit, D. F. (1989). Effects of a comprehensive program for teenage parents: Five years after project redirection. *Family Planning Perspectives, 21,* 164-169.

Polit, D. F., & Kahn, J. R. (1985). Project Redirection: Evaluation of a comprehensive program for disadvantaged teenage mothers. *Family Planning Perspectives, 17,* 150-155.

Pool, J. S., & Pool, D. I. (1978). *Contraception and health care among young Canadian women.* Ottawa: Carleton University.

Presser, H. B. (1978). Age at menarche, sociosexual behavior, and fertility. *Social Biology, 25,* 94-101.

Roberts, D. F., & Dann, T. C. (1967). Influences on menarcheal age in girls in a Welsh college. *British Journal of Preventive Social Medicine, 21,* 170-176.

Rona, R., & Pereira, G. (1974). Factors that influence age of menarche in girls in Santiago, Chile. *Human Biology, 46,* 33-42.

Rosoff, J. I. (1989). Sex education in the schools: Policies and practice. *Family Planning Perspectives, 21,* 52-54.

Sadler, L. S., & Catrone, C. (1983). The adolescent parent: A dual development crisis. *Journal of Adolescent Health Care, 4,* 100-105.

Schofield, M. (1965). *The sexual behavior of young people.* Boston: Little, Brown.

Schorr, L. B. (1985). *Within our reach: Breaking the cycle of disadvantage.* New York: Doubleday.

Shah, F., Zelnik, M., & Kantner, J. F. (1975). Unprotected intercourse among unwed teenagers. *Family Planning Perspectives, 7,* 39-44.

Short, R. V. (1976). The evolution of human reproduction. *Proceedings of the Royal Society, 195,* 3-24.

Silber, T. J. (1985). Adolescent sexuality: Developmental and ethical issues. In Pan American Health Organization (PAHO), *The health of adolescents and youths in the Americas* (Scientific Publication No. 489) (pp. 87-94). Washington, DC: PAHO.

Silverman, J., Torres, A., & Forrest, J. D. (1987). Barriers to contraceptive services. *Family Planning Perspectives, 19,* 94-102.

Simon, W., & Gagnon, J. H. (1986). Sexual scripts: Permanence and change. *Archives of Sexual Behavior, 15,* 97-120.

Simon, W., & Gagnon, J. H. (1987). A sexual scripts approach. In J. H. Geer & W. T. O'Donahue (Eds.), *Theories of human sexuality* (pp. 363-383). New York: Plenum.

Singh, S., Torres, A., & Forrest, J. D. (1985). The need for prenatal care in the United States: Evidence from the 1980 National Natality Survey. *Family Planning Perspectives, 17,* 118-124.

Smith, D. S. (1978). The dating of the American sexual revolution: Evidence and interpretation. In M. Gordon (Ed.), *The American family in social historical perspective* (2nd ed., pp. 426-438). New York: St. Martin's.

Smith, E. A. (1989). A biosocial model of adolescent sexual behavior. In G. R. Adams, T. Gullotta, & R. Montemayor (Eds.), *Biology of adolescent behavior and development* (pp. 143-167). Newbury Park, CA: Sage.

Smith, E. A., & Udry, J. R. (1985). Coital and non-coital sexual behaviors of white and black adolescents. *American Journal of Public Health, 75,* 1200-1203.

Smith, E. A., Udry, J. R., & Morris, N. M. (1985). Pubertal development and friends: A biosocial explanation of adolescent sexual behavior. *Journal of Health and Social Behavior, 26,* 183-192.

Smith, E. A., Zabin, L. S., & Hirsch, M. B. (1985, November). *Young teens, their mothers, and communication about sex: Do moms and kids agree?* Paper presented at the meeting of the American Public Health Association, Washington, DC.

Smith, T. W. (1991). Adult sexual behavior in 1989: Number of partners, frequency of intercourse and risk of AIDS. *Family Planning Perspectives, 23,* 102-107.

Sonenstein, F. L. (1986). Risking paternity: Sex and contraception among adolescent males. In A. B. Elster & M. E. Lamb (Eds.), *Adolescent fatherhood* (pp. 31-52). Hillsdale, NJ: Lawrence Erlbaum.

Sonenstein, F. L., Pleck, J. H., & Ku, L. C. (1989). Sexual activity, condom use and AIDS awareness among adolescent males. *Family Planning Perspectives, 21,* 152-158.

Sonenstein, F. L., Pleck, J. H., & Ku, L. C. (1991). Levels of sexual activity among adolescent males in the United States. *Family Planning Perspectives, 23,* 162-167.

Sorensen, R. C. (1973). *Adolescent sexuality in contemporary America.* New York: World.

Spanier, G. (1975). Sexualization and premarital sexual behavior. *Family Coordinator,* *24,* 33-41.

Strobino, D. M. (1987). The health and medical consequences of adolescent sexuality and pregnancy: A review of the literature. In S. L. Hofferth & C. D. Hayes (Eds.), *Risking the future* (Vol. 2, pp. 93-122). Washington, DC: National Academy Press.

Tanner, J. M. (1962). *Growth at adolescence.* London: Blackwell.

Tietze, C. (1978). Teenage pregnancies: Looking ahead to 1984. *Family Planning Perspectives, 10,* 205-207.

Udry, J. R. (1979). Age at menarche, at first intercourse, and at first pregnancy. *Journal of Biosocial Science, 11,* 433-441.

Udry, J. R., Billy, J.O.G., Morris, N. M., Groff, T. R., & Raj, M. H. (1985). Serum androgenic hormones motivate sexual behavior in boys. *Fertility and Sterility, 43,* 90-94.

Udry, J. R., & Cliquet, R. L. (1982). A cross-cultural examination of the relationship between ages at menarche, marriage, and first birth. *Demography, 19,* 53-63.

Udry, J. R., Talbert, L. M., & Morris, N. M. (1986). Biosocial foundations for adolescent female sexuality. *Demography, 23,* 217-230.

Upchurch, D. M., & McCarthy, J. L. (1990). The timing of a first birth and high school completion. *American Sociological Review, 55,* 224-234.

U.S. Congress, Office of Technology Assessment. (1991). *Adolescent health: Volume 1. Summary and policy options* (OTA-H-468). Washington, DC: Government Printing Office.

Werner, E. E. (1985). Stress and protective factors in children's lives. In A. R. Nicol (Ed.), *Longitudinal studies in child psychology and psychiatry* (pp. 335-356). New York: John Wiley.

Werner, E. E. (1986). A longitudinal study of perinatal risk. In D. C. Farran & J. D. McKinney (Eds.), *Risk in longitudinal development.* New York: Academic Press.

Werner, E. E., & Smith, R. S. (1982). *Vulnerable but invincible. A longitudinal study of resilient children and youth.* New York: McGraw-Hill.

Winter, L., & Breckenmaker L. C. (1991). Tailoring family planning services to the special needs of adolescents. *Family Planning Perspectives, 23,* 24-35.

Zabin, L. S. (1979). *Pregnancy risk to adolescent girls in early years of intercourse.* Unpublished doctoral dissertation, Johns Hopkins University, Baltimore.

Zabin, L. S. (1981). The impact of early use of prescription contraceptives on reducing premarital teenage pregnancies. *Family Planning Perspectives, 13,* 72-74.

Zabin, L. S. (1984). The association between smoking and sexual behavior among teens in U.S. contraceptive clinics. *American Journal of Public Health, 73,* 261-263.

Zabin, L. S. (1990). Adolescent pregnancy: The clinician's role in intervention. *Journal of General Internal Medicine, 5*(September/October Suppl.), S81-S88.

Zabin, L. S., & Clark, S. D., Jr. (1981). Why they delay: A study of teenage family planning clinic patients. *Family Planning Perspectives, 13,* 205-217.

Zabin, L. S., Hardy, J. B., Smith, E. A., & Hirsch, M. B. (1986). Substance use and its relation to sexual activity among inner-city adolescents. *Journal of Adolescent Health Care, 7,* 320-331.

Zabin, L. S., Hardy, J. B., Streett, R., & King, T. M. (1984). A school-, hospital- and university-based adolescent pregnancy prevention program: A cooperative design for service and research. *Journal of Reproductive Medicine, 29,* 421-426.

Zabin, L. S., & Hirsch, M. B. (1988). *Evaluation of pregnancy prevention programs in the school context.* Lexington, MA: D. C. Heath.

Zabin, L. S., Hirsch, M. B., & Boscia, J. A. (1990). Differential characteristics of adolescent pregnancy test patients: Abortion, childbearing and negative test groups. *Journal of Adolescent Health Care, 11,* 107-113.

Zabin, L. S., Hirsch, M. B., & Emerson, M. R. (1989). When urban adolescents choose abortion: Effects on education, psychological status and subsequent pregnancy. *Family Planning Perspectives, 21,* 248-255.

Zabin, L. S., Hirsch, M. B., Raymond, E., & Emerson, M. R. (in press). To whom do girls talk about their pregnancies? Urban adolescents' communication with responsible adults. *Family Planning Perspectives, 24,* 148-154, 173.

Zabin, L. S., Hirsch, M. B., Smith, E. A., & Hardy, J. B. (1984). Adolescent sexual attitudes and behavior: Are they consistent? *Family Planning Perspectives, 16,* 181-185.

Zabin, L. S., Hirsch, M. B., Smith, E. A., Smith, M., Emerson, M. R., King, T. M., Streett, R., & Hardy, J. B. (1988). The Baltimore pregnancy prevention program for urban teenagers. 2. What did it cost? *Family Planning Perspectives, 20,* 188-192.

Zabin, L. S., Hirsch, M. B., Smith, E. A., Streett, R., & Hardy, J. B. (1986a). Adolescent pregnancy-prevention program. A model for research and evaluation. *Journal of Adolescent Health Care, 7,* 77-87.

Zabin, L. S., Hirsch, M. B., Smith, E. A., Streett, R., & Hardy, J. B. (1986b). Evaluation of a pregnancy prevention program for urban teenagers. *Family Planning Perspectives, 18,* 119-126.

Zabin, L. S., Hirsch, M. B., Streett, R., Emerson, M. R., Smith, M., Hardy, J. B., & King, T. M. (1988). The Baltimore pregnancy prevention program for urban teenagers. 1. How did it work? *Family Planning Perspectives, 20,* 182-187.

Zabin, L. S., Kantner, J. K., & Zelnik, M. (1979). The risk of adolescent pregnancy in the first months of intercourse. *Family Planning Perspectives, 11,* 215-222.

Zabin, L. S., Smith, E. A., Hirsch, M. B., & Hardy, J. B. (1986). Ages of physical maturation and first intercourse in black teenage males and females. *Demography, 23,* 595-605.

Zabin, L. S., Stark, H. A., & Emerson M. R. (1991). Reasons for delay in contraceptive clinic utilization: Adolescent clinic and non-clinic populations compared. *Journal of Adolescent Health Care, 12,* 225-232.

Zabin, L. S., & Streett, R. (1991). The crisis of teen pregnancy and an empirically tested model for pregnancy prevention. In A. R. Roberts (Ed.), *Contemporary perspectives on crisis intervention and prevention* (pp. 240-255). Englewood Cliffs, NJ: Prentice Hall.

Zabin, L. S., Wong, R., Weinick, R. M., & Emerson, M. R. (1992). Dependency in urban black families following the birth of an adolescent's child. *Journal of Marriage and the Family, 54,* 496-507.

Zacharias, L., Wurtman, R. J., & Schatzoff, M. (1970). Sexual maturation of contemporary American girls. *American Journal of Obstetrics and Gynecology, 108,* 833-840.

Zelnik, M., & Kantner, J. F. (1973). Sex and contraception among unmarried teenagers. In D. F. Westoff (Ed.), *Toward the end of growth* (pp. 7-18). Englewood Cliffs, NJ: Prentice Hall.

Zelnik, M., & Kantner, J. F. (1977). Sexual and contraceptive experience of young unmarried women in the United States, 1976 and 1971. *Family Planning Perspectives, 9,* 55-71.

Zelnik, M., & Kantner, J. F. (1980). Sexual activity, contraceptive use and pregnancy among metropolitan-area teenagers: 1971-1979. *Family Planning Perspectives, 12,* 230-237.

Zelnik, M., Kantner, J. F., & Ford, K. (1981). *Sex and pregnancy in adolescence.* Beverly Hills, CA: Sage.

Zelnik, M., Kim, Y. J., & Kantner, J. F. (1979). Probabilities of intercourse among U.S. teenage women, 1971 and 1976. *Family Planning Perspectives, 11,* 177-183.

Zelnik, M., Koenig, M. A., & Kim, Y. J. (1984). Source of prescription contraceptives and subsequent pregnancy among women. *Family Planning Perspectives, 16,* 6-13.

Zelnik, M., & Shah, F. K. (1983). First intercourse among young Americans. *Family Planning Perspectives, 15,* 64-70.

INDEX

ABOUT THE AUTHORS

Laurie Schwab Zabin, Ph.D., is Associate Professor in the Department of Population Dynamics at the Johns Hopkins School of Hygiene and Public Health. After long experience in population and family planning, she is now a researcher in reproductive health, focusing especially on adolescent sexual behavior, pregnancy, and childbearing and their programmatic and policy implications. Formerly Chair of the Board of Directors of the Alan Guttmacher Institute and the Population Section of the American Public Health Association, on whose Governing Council she currently serves, she also serves on the Adolescent Health Care Committee of the American College of Obstetrics and Gynecology.

Sarah C. Hayward BNSc, MPH, is currently a Project Coordinator with the Teaching Health Unit of the Hamilton-Wentworth Department of Public Health Services, Ontario, Canada. Prior to entering the field of public health she studied English and Philosophy in England, then went to Canada for her professional training at Queen's University, Kingston, Ontario. Work in various aspects of reproductive health care led to an interest in health policy and population dynamics. She completed a Master of Public Health degree at John Hopkins University in 1991, and subsequently worked with Laurie Schwab Zabin on the development of this publication.